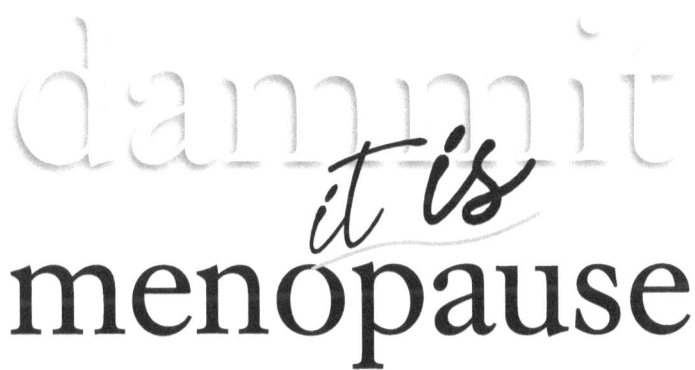

Meditations for Women to
Achieve Clarity and Confidence
Beyond Their Wildest Dreams

# Sally Bartlett

volume one

**Dammit ... *It IS* Menopause!**
Meditations for Women to Achieve Clarity and
Confidence Beyond Their Wildest Dreams, volume 1
Sally Bartlett
© Copyright 2021
ALL RIGHTS RESERVED

With certain exceptions, no part of this book may be reproduced in any written,
electronic, recording, or photocopying form without written permission
of the publisher or author. The exceptions would be in the case of brief
quotations embodied in critical articles or reviews and pages where permission
is specifically granted in writing by the author or publisher and where
authorship/source is acknowledged in the quoted materials.

Published by Ginger Books Press
website: SallyBartlett.com
ISBN print: 978-1-7358785-1-5
ISBN eBook: 978-1-7358785-2-2
ISBN audio: 978-1-7358785-3-9

Library of Congress Control Number: 2020920420
Editors: Margaret Ireland, Judith Briles
Book Shepherd: Judith Briles
Cover, interior and eBook design: F + P Graphic Design, FPGD.com

First Edition
Printed in the United States

WOMEN'S HEALTH   |   MENOPAUSE   |   MEDITATIONS

*To all women*

*who are at any stage*

*of menopause.*

*You are not alone.*

# Author's Note

***Dammit ... It IS Menopause!*** I was SO hoping it was just a hangnail or something. This was my first response when the symptoms began at age 45.

Apparently book titles are super important. Who knew? This being my first book, I had no idea. Never gave it much thought. Having said that, I'd like to give some backstory on mine. My original title was *How to Avoid Basketball Stomach.* I have maintained a 35-lb. weight loss without dieting for over 30 years. I consider myself a former volume eater and exercise bulimic who has recovered from disordered eating for more than three decades now. This healthy homeostasis doesn't come without work. The secret to being where I am is my commitment to PIES. Got your attention? I am referring to my commitment to consistent, daily self-care on multiple levels:

- Physically
- Intellectually
- Emotionally
- Spiritually

If you are like me, there's nothing like a food reference to get your attention. A component that set the foundation for my daily self-care, PIES was loving my body exactly the way it was at my heaviest weight, all those years ago. Close to 200 lbs.

As I said, I lost my weight without dieting. Yes, I just said that. I recognize I am somewhat of an anomaly, given today's diet-focused culture. But after years of unsuccessful dieting attempts from my teens through my early twenties, I finally realized I would not find success in dieting. Wait. Let's stop here to define "diet success." My definition of diet success is losing the weight ***and keeping it off for over 10 years.*** If any diet can offer me that, I would call it successful. Given that definition, I've yet to find a successful diet. Not only are diets unsuccessful, in most cases they create an unhealthy binge/fast eating behavior, which perpetuates a destructive emotional shame spiral that worsens over time.

By the time I was 24 years old, I had tried every diet available at the time. Trust me. I am quite thorough. I was miserable, frustrated, discouraged, depressed, and exhausted. Not to mention I weighed even more than I had when the dieting began. On top of that, I still loathed everything about myself. If I discovered anything in my years of personal diet research, it was my four Value Epiphanies:

1. Sustained daily commitment to living in and loving a healthy-sized body (determined by me) for optimal quality of life and aging, PIES.

2. Living free from food obsession and self-loathing.

3. Dieting will never be the route to get there. Ever.

4. Sharing this message with as many women as possible so they too may live a Big Amazing Life as I do.

Knowing my body-dysmorphic, disordered eating history, you can imagine I come from a family where undue importance was placed on looks and body size. I continue working to dismantle that mentality to this day. Progress … not perfection. That said, when I began my peri-menopausal journey in my mid-40s, my biggest fear was gaining a disproportional amount of weight in my midsection. My thinking was, "I have spent ten years loving living in this body. I'll be damned if I'm gonna lose it now." At 60 years of age now, I look back and see this as clear evidence that remnants of my original body-dysmorphia mindset still lingered. There is always work to do.

I wrote *Dammit* over the course of 15 years, from age 45 to 60. During this time, I have come to a new acceptance and love of my amazing aging body. I realized that I no longer feared what my body shape would become. I returned to my original Value Epiphanies, renewing my commitment to live in and love my healthy-sized body for optimal quality of life and aging, PIES. I let go of fears and judgments about the shape of my body, and I let go of derogatory nicknames for parts of my body, such as "Basketball."

So began the quest for a new book title. I wanted a title that was more reflective of my successful aging evolution, a title that reflected my shifted, more accepting self-narrative. I spent time contemplating.

• • •

First, I looked to my fitness, wellness, and menopause coaching practice for book title ideas. I am known as the Dean of Varsity Menopause, so it seemed natural to call my book *Meditations for Varsity Menopause.* When I proposed the new title, the Varsity Menopause concept was met with wrinkled noses, and was swiftly vetoed by people who knew far more about book naming than I. Some people immediately got me and loved it. Others responded simply with a long, thoughtful pause.

People ask me, "What do you mean by *Varsity* menopause? What could varsity and menopause possibly have in common?" And "Why the dean title?"

## Inspiration for VARSITY

Where did my inspiration for "Varsity" come from? We all know life can be hard. Persevering through life's ups and downs can be daunting. I deal with depression many mornings and insomnia some nights. Sometimes I just want to give up, especially when it comes to menopause and aging. But I will never give up. I always want to live, despite the challenges I face. Whenever my friend Cordelia and I face unexpected challenges, we always exclaim, "Thank You, God, for this growth opportunity!" I want to live, no matter what.

How do I carry on? What's my secret? The secret to successful aging is getting out of myself and connecting with other humans. We are not meant to live in isolation. As women, we are not meant to compete with each other. We are meant to connect with each other. I am grateful to have a circle of supportive friends. We support each other by listening to each other's struggles. We support each other by acknowledging each other's triumphs—big and small.

One day years ago, I chatted on the phone with my friend, Cordelia, about my accomplishments for that day. I had finally completed a task that had been on my to-do list for way longer than I had wanted. It had been driving me crazy. I don't even remember what the thing was on this occasion. It wasn't anything big like earning a college degree or cleaning out the entire garage. It was more on a par with cleaning out the vegetable drawer in the fridge for the first time in six years. Whatever it was, Cordelia responded in her typical deadpan, mock-serious monotone voice, "That's Varsity, lady." I simultaneously felt heard and validated, and we both roared with laughter. It stuck. Ever since that day, whenever either of us deems that the other has accomplished something impressive, no matter how big or small, the other will enthusiastically exclaim, "That's Varsity!"

Akin to awesome, Varsity is exponentially more powerful. Awesome is a little overused anyway, if you ask me. The Varsity proclamation is a way that we acknowledge each other and build each other up. It's a way we show support for each other. In lifting others up, I lift myself up as well. Plus, I have to say, I feel pretty good about myself when someone tells me I'm Varsity.

I've found that the Varsity message is universally understood and appreciated. Sometimes I strike up a conversation in the grocery store checkout line with a stranger. The person may tell me some random thing s/he has discovered or accomplished. I will validate with a resounding, "That's Varsity!" It's easy to see from the sparkle in the person's eyes and the smile spreading across his/her face that the meaning is understood. The world needs more of that message.

## Inspiration for DEAN

During that same season of book title contemplation, my son graduated from high school and prepared to leave home for college. I knew my job title of 18 years was about to shift radically, but I had no idea what it would be shifting to. I knew it would be a challenge for me to pivot from my coveted role as single mother of an only child. I knew there would be a few extra hours in the day to spend on things other than parenting. I was more than a little nervous about what that was going to look like. The heat was on to prepare myself for my new life in a new role. I took the challenge head-on and began listening intently to every entrepreneurial podcast I could find. Per my usual intense self-diagnosed, gently-OCD style, I took notes and created folders corresponding to podcasters who inspired me most. Gradually, a vision for a scaled version of my existing coaching practice took shape. There was a mixture of feelings ranging from paralyzing fear to excited, unknown euphoria.

Meanwhile, THE day came. While my son attended his college students' orientation, I attended mine. There I sat in the parents' orientation, supposedly learning how to use the parent portal. But my mind wandered as I silently wondered what the empty nest was going to be like for me as a single parent of an only child, whom I gave birth to at the age of 40. This kid … we are close. I later learned that some of my friends secretly expected I would disintegrate upon his departure (thanks for that). And in fact, they expected that neither my son nor I would fare too well without each other. They couldn't have been more wrong. We have both thrived beyond our wildest dreams. But I digress.

Suddenly I snapped out of my internal catastrophizing, crying, future-tripping session in time to hear that the Dean of Students would be the next speaker. For some reason, I perked up at this title. Dean. What was the job of a dean of an organization? To promote development. To enhance success. To facilitate a respectful, diverse and inclusive environment. To provide direct support for successful navigation for a season of life. Before I knew it, I was snapping photos of the slide show with my cell. This was precisely describing the role I have played for my clients for years. Suddenly it hit me ... I am a dean. I am the Dean of Varsity Menopause.

I invite you to join me on your aging journey. I strive to act as the dean to help you see it as a Varsity menopause experience. The best is yet to come.

I have been exactly where you are right now. Perimenopause and menopause are not something that you would have added to your "to-do" list when you had your first period. After all, a young girl most likely doesn't have those words in her vocabulary. But you and certainly I do several decades later ... and I wished I hadn't had to learn them the hard way.

*Dammit ... It IS Menopause!* is me talking to you and sharing with you. And yes, pulling out my hair and crying with you. I've been there ... wish I hadn't ... and yet I survived.

Originally, I planned to write a book of meditations for pregnant women. When I resurfaced for air after having had my first child, I really wanted to have another baby. Apparently, the Universe had other plans. Lo and behold, at 45, and much to my chagrin, my body seemed to have other plans besides childbirth.

Yes, the "M" word reared its ugly head. To embrace this new chapter in my life, even though I hadn't given my female body permission for this unwelcome "chapter," I've compiled a book of meditations for perimenopausal and menopausal women. More than a decade and a half later, I can honestly say I have embraced menopause and the discoveries and freedom that accompany it. And I am flourishing in what I call my *Varsity Way.*

*Dammit ... it IS Menopause!* is a book of essays, meditations and prayers that are primarily addressed to God, along with calls to action and reflections. It encompasses the journeys of several women of varying ages, in many stages of perimenopause ... and my own. I began writing because I was so distraught and uncomfortable with the changes in my personality, my thinking, my confidence, my body, and basically everything about myself as a result of perimenopause that hit me around the age of 45.

At the onset, I felt terribly alone, and feared I was losing my mind. What you have before your eyes is meant to be a lighthearted, yet solutions-oriented, spiritual resource so you don't have to feel alone like I did! You will laugh at times. In fact, it's recommended and extremely important. It is meant to open the door for women to communicate and comfort each other during what could be a potentially trying time.

*To protect the privacy of the women whose stories are shared herein, I refer to all of them as "Cordelia," after my Great-Aunt Cordy (1900-1985). This book is about self-acceptance, and my Aunt Cordy was someone from whom I received unconditional acceptance at a young age while going through a challenging period of my life.*

Although I mostly use God when referring to a higher power, you can certainly substitute anything that works for your concept of a Power greater than yourself. Throughout my journaling, I often reach out to God (aka Big Love) in desperation, and I sometimes get responses … some profound and some humorous.

The prayers, reflections, and calls to action are meant as suggestions to help you find solutions to situations you may be experiencing.

You can read the entries in order, a day at a time, or skip around, based on what you are experiencing. As I have learned from my own experiences and the many stories shared with me by other women, hormone level changes can be experienced in many ways and at all ages. Just because you are at a certain level hormonally, it doesn't mean your life is over! Far from it.

You have so much more living to do! And many people to live it with. Commit to bloom where you are planted and join my Varsity Menopause Team!

My Heart messages to you:
Don't waste another second being unkind to yourself or doubting yourself or playing small.

You are being prepared to receive all the love and joy your heart can hold.

Take the time to invest in yourself. You're worth it!

— Sally

PART I

# Early Awareness

# My Story

*Around the age of 10,* my mother put me on my first diet. She had only the best of intentions, but looking back, I realized that my weight had made *her* uncomfortable. I had been fine with it. The body that made her uncomfortable was functioning just as it needed to be in preparation for the onset of puberty. Years later, I have made peace with my cherished anorexic mom, knowing that she loved me as much as a mother could love a child, and was merely passing on what was taught to her at my age. I am grateful for having the right mom for me.

Thus began my 14-year spiral deep into the world of what I refer to as "diet mentality," which included endless dieting accompanied by dangerously rapid weight fluctuation and progressive weight gain, perfectionism, compulsive exercising, people-pleasing and negative self-talk in an effort to feel good enough and thin enough to be lovable. You name it, there was not a diet I hadn't tried between 1969 and 1984. Trust me on this. No need to name them.

My primary focus throughout college was compulsive eating and dieting while I was earning my BA in psychology from the University of California at Berkeley. I considered myself a relatively intelligent person, but it took me another six years to confront my situation head-on and act.

Finally, in my late 20s, I made radical lifestyle changes to my physical, intellectual, emotional, and spiritual components. I made peace with my body and I made peace with food. I lost about 35 pounds for the last time, God willing. This time, my primary objective went much deeper than merely taking the weight off. I aspired to *keep* the weight off, long-term. Having been completely ensconced in diet mentality for well over a decade by then, I had a lot of work to do to heal. I soon learned that to experience lifelong weight loss maintenance, my participation needed to be on multiple levels. This was going to be much more than merely a journey about *physical* recovery. I slowly lost the weight at the rate of about two pounds per MONTH. And once the weight was off, then the hard work began. Yes, my body was now officially "right-sized," but there was so much more to it than the size of my physical body.

As a fitness professional and former bulimic exerciser, I knew all about staying in "fit" physical condition. What I didn't know was how to stay in fit *spiritual* condition, in fit *emotional* condition, or even in fit *mental* condition.

To maintain my new body, I needed these three other components. I had lost the weight so many times before, only to gain it, and more weight, back. This time I was determined to go to any lengths—to do whatever it took. Around the age of 28, I embarked on an entirely new journey that I am still (usually) happily on today. Even through pregnancy, I remained in what I called a right-sized body and mind.

> I have not owned a scale in 30 years. I get on the scale backwards if a doctor asks me to weigh in.

Then in my 40s, hormonal shift happened. I basically had to recalibrate my entire lifestyle—physically, intellectually, emotionally, and spiritually—that had worked for me for over a decade to address the extreme symptoms that accompanied these shifts. My entire personality changed. Would I and could I rise to the occasion? I was in total denial—menopause … surely, not me!

*Dammit … it IS Menopause!* is the journey of my struggles through this phase of womanhood. I invented many tips and techniques to keep myself on track—and I am gladly sharing these with you. This is a serious subject.

Paralleling this is an issue that I have been dealing with seemingly my entire life: my daily decisions regarding imperfect healthy food choices and amounts. I've let my quirky humor loose, scattered here and there for some levity. And I'm sure you will relate to some of my predicaments. We women are comforted in knowing we are not alone, right?!

Even through pregnancy at 40, perimenopause and beyond, I have remained in what I call a right-sized body and mind. A body I can do business with. A body I love the hell out of.

I have been fully menopausal for over 10 years now. At my annual wellness exam, I stand on the office scale backward and only ask the nurse every other year what I weigh. I have not owned a scale in 30 years. And during my entire pregnancy, when the doctor wanted to document my weight, I got on the scale backwards. Not until six months after my son was born did I ask what my weight was. I learned that my weight the day before I delivered my child at 40 years of age was still lower than my top weight in my 20s. I continue to feel good and my clothes keep fitting, year after year.

It is not about the weight. The weight is a barometer of what I am eating, and what I am eating is a barometer of how well I am staying current with my feelings.

If you have read to this point, chances are these thoughts and feelings resonate with you. I wholeheartedly invite you to join me in these pages as I share all my secrets about how I live a Varsity life: physically, intellectually, emotionally, and spiritually. Come on this journey to discover your Big Amazing Life. It's waiting for you!

Through perimenopause and beyond, I have remained in a right-sized body and mind, wholly determined by me.

It's your turn … I have a quiz for you. It only requires a "yes" or "no" response. It will take a few minutes to complete. Answer where you are right now. You could be perimenopausal, in the heart of menopause, or postmenopausal.

## The Varsity Menopause Quiz

- Do you feel that you've lost your way with the onset of hormonal shift?
- Do you dislike your body image and have disliked your body all your life?
- Have you ever thought "I'll be loveable when I lose 10 pounds"?
- Do you understand that preexisting body image issues are exacerbated during menopause?

- Has your previously healthy body image deteriorated with the onset of your hormonal shift?
- Are any deep negative self-talk barriers keeping you from reaching your true potential?
- Do you repeatedly allow yourself to be held back by believing your self-limiting beliefs (that are untrue)?
- Have you lost sight of your "normal" life as you knew it?
- Are you grieving the end of childbearing years, end of "youth," end of pulchritude (sensuality, womanhood), plus other things you may be surprised to discover but are too afraid to explore?
- Do you fear being deemed obsolete by others in your life, or do you feel that way about yourself?
- Are you experiencing overwhelming physiological symptoms, such as hot flashes, vaginal dryness, mood swings, erratic periods, cramps all the time, breast pain, waking in the middle of the night, inability to stay asleep or go back to sleep, body odor, dry skin, itching that wakes you up, night sweats, hair loss (but may not have wanted to connect the dots)?
- Are you suddenly more forgetful than ever in your life?
- Have you experienced "brain fog" – trouble finding the right word you want to say?

- Have you experienced crying jags that are uncontrollable, bursting into tears for no reason?
- Are there times when you feel your identity is challenged?
- Are there times that your self-esteem plummets?
- Do you ever think you are going crazy?
- Are there days where you don't recognize yourself?
- Have levels of self-doubt surfaced?
- Do you feel depressed?
- Is there a disinterest in sex, or has intercourse become painful? (usually due to vaginal dryness)
- Do (or did) you fear that your life is over?
- Do you fear you will not be loveable anymore?
- Do you feel a decreased energy level?
- Are your joints sore?
- Is exercise not as enjoyable as it has been for years?
- Have you noticed a change in your body shape, even though you are consuming the same healthy diet that has kept you fit for years?
- Do you have a belief in the shame-based body culture we live in that is not serving you?

If you answered mostly YES to the above questions, you are in the right place.

*Get ready to regain clarity and conviction about your identity and your purpose in life.*

It's time to improve your self-acceptance, body-confidence, and self-esteem, both during and after the advent of hormonal shift. Along the journey with me, here's what else happens:

✓ Develop a more current self-image with respect to aging, whether you have had self-image issues all your life or issues are just now arising for the first time with the onset of perimenopause.

✓ Sleep better and regain interest in sensual pleasure.

✓ Break free from long-standing negative self-talk barriers to smash limiting beliefs.

✓ Become the open-minded woman who can reach goals previously unattainable.

✓ Feel more loveable, courageous, willing to try things you've avoided.

✓ Regain your sense of a "normal" life.

✓ Reignite passion for your Big Amazing Life with potential and stop living a tiny, closed-in life.

✓ Learn to identify and process feelings; increase emotional literacy.

✓ Improve Emotional Regulation by getting current and staying current with your feelings via my suggested calls to action in this book.

✓ Learn new ways of living where you stay in touch with feelings and reignite and challenge your intellect.

Get out of isolation to create a new story about your body and your life that undoes shame, isolation and competition while surrounding yourself with supportive, like-minded women.

You will get immense comfort in knowing you're not the only one going through this, and be able to speak openly about issues many women are afraid of or uncomfortable talking about. Does that sound like you? It's time to break free from the diet mindset of exercising to "work off" the most recent bout of spontaneous eating.

I'm excited for you to right-size your mindset around exercising for the purpose of disease prevention and healthy aging, cardiovascular health, muscle strength, bone strength, balance, fighting depression, sleeping better, fluid, pain-free movement, and adding to your energy levels. I'm honored to share my insights and experiences as I wove my way through the menopause maze. Are you ready to ignite your passions and embrace this amazing new you? Would you like more peace and confidence and to be kinder to yourself?

And are you ready for optimism to flow through you about aging and menopause, and being a woman?

# 1
# This Can't Be Happening to Me

Looking back, my first realization that something unfamiliar was going on with me was when I was about 45 years old. I was crying more than my usual PMS (premenstrual syndrome) amount ... sobbing. I called my friend Cordelia, saying, "I don't know why I keep crying so much today. I don't feel like myself."

What was happening to me? I was in the midst of choosing which kindergarten to send our son to in seven months. I know that's big, but the volume of tears that were flooding my ducts just didn't seem to match the intensity of the circumstance. I felt this strange urge to call my son's preschool teacher to discuss my options. From the phone I told her, between sobs, I wanted to speak to her, and asked if she was available. I had never cried in front of her, so she probably thought I was dying or something.

She offered to see me right away. When I arrived at her classroom, the floodgates were open. This volume of crying alone was unusual for me. But doing so in front of someone was even more out of character. It … wasn't … me. Even so, having talked things out, I left her feeling much better. Time passed and I forgot about that day as I went on to the next things in life.

> Dear God,
> Help me remember that it's okay to cry. That it feels quite healing. Remind me to trust that You have a plan for me. Even though it seems like I don't understand what's going on with me and like it's the end of the world. That You want to use me in a powerful way, even though I don't know what it is yet.

# 2

## Am I Losing It?

*In the weeks following the crying jag episode*, I exhibited several other traits that were abnormal for me. I misplaced my keys. Except for one time at age 16 when I locked my car keys in the trunk, I am not the key-losing type. On top of that, I left the house without my purse more than once. This is SO not me, and what's more, I was on a trip to purchase one of my favorite things—frozen yogurt. I do not think I have ever left home without my purse prior to this time … EVER!

> Dear God,
> What is going on with me? Why am I doing all these things that are so out of character for me? Please give me patience and self-compassion as I embrace and explore this new place in my life … gentle, gentle.

# 3

## FEELING OLD, FORGETFUL AND OVERWHELMED: MAKING MISTAKES, EXPERIENCING A DIMINISHED ABILITY TO FOCUS

*I made the mistake* of looking at my bare arms in the distorted reflection of the car window today. Bad idea: I feel really old. As if that weren't enough, my four-year-old son keeps getting frustrated with me when I don't complete sentences because I have forgotten what I was talking about mid-sentence. Several times lately I have put on the wrong turn signal while driving. Things that used to seem insignificant now seem overwhelming and I just want to go to bed. I frequently forget where I was going, what I was doing, or whom I was calling, all for no apparent reason.

Dear God,
I feel so frustrated. What's going on? Please guide me. Give me the ability to embrace "what is" for today.

# 4
# Is PMS Supposed to Last 3 Weeks?

*Another early perimenopausal (PM) awareness* was that my state of PMS-ness seemed endless. We are talking sore boobs, acne, and cramps, to name a few. I even entertained crazy fantasies. Any PMS woman knows what I'm talking about. Whereas I used to be a little cranky for the 3–7 days prior to my period, now I had a full-blown Murder-Death-Kill—aka MDK from *Demolition Man,* 1993 sci-fi action film—attitude for at least three weeks prior to the big day.

> Dear God,
> What is going on? I don't like it. Help me trust You to get me through this uncertain time.

# 5

# So Tired of "Sporting a String"

*Around the time* these new awarenesses about my body began, one of the first things that I noticed was my periods began to last much longer than I was accustomed to. When I have my period, my husband thinks it's funny to call it "sporting a string." Ha ha ha—NOT. Anyway, whatever—the point is, it gets really tiring after eight days or so. I constantly feel gross and like I need a shower, no matter how often I bathe.

About two months after the crying jag with the preschool teacher, my period lasted a full 21 days. As my periods generally last four days MAX, this was an all-time record, not to mention a pain in the … string.

On one visit to my OB/Gyn, she told me a little trick to shorten my period. She told me that if I take ibuprofen around the clock according to the directions on the bottle as soon as there's even a hint that my period is about to begin, it will **decrease volume and duration by about 50-percent.**

Of course, I tried it the very next month and sure enough, it worked for me! Remember, I am not a doctor. This is just what happened to me.

But guess what's in every medicine chest in our house now?

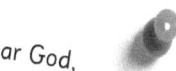

Dear God,

I feel scared and uncomfortable because a lot of weird things are happening to me. I don't understand it, I don't like it, and I did not give my permission for any of this. Please help me to remember that this, too, shall pass. Help me to trust that this is supposed to be happening and that I will live through it.

# 6

# Precious OCD Girl Searches in Vain for Menstrual Cycle Patterns

I love patterns. I especially love to analyze, chart, and graph anything that pertains to bodily functions. When my son was born, I had difficulty getting into a routine with breastfeeding, so I composed a table to record my son's bodily functions regarding his feeding frequency and duration. In a way, charting relaxes and comforts me. It enables me to let go of things a little.

So naturally I tried to find a pattern to my menstrual cycles … impossible. I would have 40-day cycles followed by 20-day cycles. I would have PMS symptoms for three weeks prior to my period, followed by a period that lasted only two days. Then it would stop for two days, then resume for two weeks. I had cramps and sore boobs before, during, and after my period. I experienced anything and everything relative to my menstrual cycle except what I had experienced for the preceding adult years of my life.

> Dear God,
> Give me the courage to embrace change. I feel scared and sad and lost. I feel as if I am floating in outer space with no anchor and absolutely no direction. Please give me strength.

# 7
# This Is the End of the World – Hair Trauma Edition

*I have naturally curly, frizzy, wavy red hair.* I was teased relentlessly as a child. When I was about 46, I discovered the flat iron, which enables me to make my hair smooth, shiny, and straight; something I have wished for my entire life. This was before chemical straightening, which I'll tell you about in another journal entry. I realized that I had become extremely attached to my flat iron, but when do you know if you have a problem with flat iron dependence?

On the morning of my son's end-of-preschool music pageant, I was alone in the house, air conditioning blasting, and mega-sized ice water within reach. I was in the hair-styling "zone," on the home stretch of blow drying—the phase just prior to ironing. Suddenly, I blew the fuse for my dryer. Annoyed, I searched the house for another operative plug. The only one in the house that worked had no mirror near it. Throwing on a bathrobe, I went outside to the circuit breaker to see what I could do. I am not the most electrically minded person. I had no luck. Presently my parents arrived to ride with me to the pageant. By then I was freaking out because besides being late, I had begun to perspire, and it was ruining my makeup. My ultra-conservative parents weren't quite sure what to make of my ranting and raving with half my hair dry and the other half in a giant clippie and wearing only a skimpy bathrobe.

Eventually I finished the hairdo using an extension cord. This is my answer to every electrical problem. I once regained the use of electricity by extending multiple extension cords between our neighbor's house and ours when we lost power because my darling husband had forgotten to pay our electric bill. But I digress.

This outburst was yet another sign to me that something was going on with me. I knew that my anxiety level exceeded what it normally would have been in this situation. What was going on?

> Dear God,
> Please make these behavior changes stop, or at least explain why they are occurring. I feel so strange. I don't feel at all like myself. What did You do with Sally? Please bring her back.

# 8

## Taking Surveys

*Akin to my love of charting,* I also love what I call "taking surveys." When I discovered I had contracted toenail fungus several years ago, I launched an informal survey among my friends about the subject. Being the recovering perfectionist I am, my initial reaction to things like this is horror and I say things like, "This must be some sort of mistake. This is not supposed to be happening to *me*." Whatever life experience I may be going through, it helps me to get into acceptance mode when I talk about it with others.

I learned that at least three of my close friends had had toenail fungus to one degree or another for years. And my good friends still wanted to be my friend when I disclosed my situation. It turned out that even my Uncle Dick was prone to it. And he had gone on to live a normal life! I guess I would, too, I realized to my relief.

So, I take surveys a lot to gain perspective and give myself permission to rejoin humanity with my fellow man.

> Dear God,
> Please help me remember I am not alone in my imperfections. Not only am I lovable and loved despite my imperfections but because of them. Thank You. I feel so much better.

# 9
# WHEN YOU'RE HOT, YOU'RE HOT... AND NOT IN A GOOD WAY: PART 1

*The next strange awareness* I had was that I seemed to be warmer than usual—*constantly*. It was the beginning of summer, so at first, I just assumed that was the reason. But then I started to perspire in weird places, like the backs of my knees and the tops of my thighs, and at weird times, like in the evening when it wasn't really that warm out anymore. And now those odd women at the gym in my Cardio Dance Party classes who always demanded the overhead fans be turned on didn't seem so odd anymore. In fact, now I would high-five them when they did so.

It was clearly time for me to do another survey. At first, I was really against holding a conversation using any "perimenopausal" vernacular. I reluctantly talked to one of my best friends, Cordelia (60), about the "F" word (hot FLASH). She assured me there would be no mistaking it if I were having a hot flash. She said it would feel like this Mount Vesuvius burning sensation coming up through me like a volcano. I had not experienced anything like that, so I breathed a sigh of relief. This perimenopause thing was just in my head. Thank God I'm not there!

> Dear God,
> I am so grateful I am NOT having hot flashes and therefore could not possibly be starting menopause. Thank You!

# 10

## When You're Hot, You're Hot: Part II

*Continuing with my body temperature survey,* I learned more than I wanted to. Another friend explained it like this: "I get this all-over warming, including sweat at the top of my head, face, neck and chest." Another said: "I feel heat suddenly, as if someone turned on the heater, and I start to sweat. And it happens at least two times a day."

I got a lot of responses to this subject. Yet another said: "All of a sudden, I feel like I have a heating pad on my back." My friend Cordelia had named two variations of hot flashes she had experienced. One was "red prickly heat" and one was "baptism by fire." Another friend jokingly refers to it as "having your own private summer." Although I hadn't experienced anything like these descriptions, I didn't think it was funny. They all sounded awful.

> Please God,
> Can't this all just be a bad dream? I don't want my own private summer. I am ready to wake up and be 23 years old again, please and thank You.

# 11

## Everyone Just F-ing Get Away From Me!

*About a month* after the first crying-jag-to-people-I-hardly-know situation, I was extremely irritated with my students at work. At the time, I was a group fitness instructor for older adults. My students ranged in age from 60 to 100 years old. They inspired me daily because they were in incredible shape, body, mind, and spirit. They loved to laugh, and they frequently hugged me, and brought me cards and food. Are you envisioning how irritating all that would be (NOT!)?

Anyway, throughout my professional life I have made it my policy not to swear at work. With my girlfriends it's another story, but at work, I am consistent about this. One day at work, something inside me just seemed to snap. I pulled one of my coworkers aside and asked in a whispering mock-scream, "DO YOU EVER JUST WANT TO YELL, 'F@#% YOU!' to your students?" She just looked at me knowingly, nodding.

Later at home, I couldn't believe I had done that. When I next returned to work, I once again pulled my coworker aside and apologized, making reference to hormones running amok (even though I was sure that couldn't be my problem because I still plan to have another baby and don't you know I am too young to be going through menopause?). She merely laughed, patted my arm, and said, "Oh, this won't be the last time that happens." What was she talking about? This was an isolated incident. Boy, was I in for a rude awakening.

> Dear God,
> Please help me be gentle with myself as this new person emerges. I don't think I like her. I feel confused and sad about it. Help me to love her through this, just as You love her.

# 12
## Critical Inner Voice Buys a Bullhorn and Works Overtime

*I have a critical voice* inside my head that talks incessantly. No, I am not psychotic, to the best of my knowledge. It's a voice that constantly shames me or "shoulds" on me.

"You *should* not have said that." "You *should* have done that." "You *should* already know how to do that." "You *should* be finished already." If I had to draw a picture of what's going on in my head, I would draw a little man riding atop a big old 1970s station wagon, carrying a bullhorn, and screaming these mean things. Would I say things like this to you? No! Would I keep people in my life who spoke to me this way? Absolutely not. Someone said S.H.A.M.E. is an acronym: Should Have Already Mastered Everything.

I have been aware of my critical inner voice for years. I have been successful in overriding the voice with a more positive voice through frequent writing exercises. However, in the past few months, the voice seems to be on steroids or something.

Luckily, also residing inside that fabulous brain of mine is a still, small voice encouraging me. The one that says, "You did the best you could in the moment," or "you handled that really well." "I know this is new for you but hang in there and you'll learn how to do it." "Keep practicing because you'll get the timing just right."

Why my inner dialogue exists in my head no longer matters to me. My main concern is getting that bullhorn out of the critical voice's hands and putting it into a compassionate voice's (CV's) hands. I write to accomplish that.

> Example of Critical Voice/Compassionate Voice Writing:
> *My Critical Voice:*
> *Dear Sally,*
> *Pull yourself together! Why can't you complete your sentences lately? Are you really college-educated? Everyone thinks you are lame.*
>
> My Compassionate Voice:
> *Dear Sally-Girl,*
> *You are amazing! I love you even though you are sometimes not able to complete sentences lately. I know you are doing the best you can. You are so very lovable just the way you are. I will help you come to terms with all this.*

*Dear God,*
*Please help me minimize my use of the word "should."*

> Dear God,
> Please let me NOT be starting PM.

# 13

## THIS CAN'T BE HAPPENING TO ME... I AM STILL SCHEDULED TO HAVE ONE MORE CHILD (A GIRL, PLEASE) & "NIGHT WARMS"

*In a phone conversation with my friend,* Cordelia (40), she told me she was informed by her doctor that she was PM. Even though I still wasn't connecting my own proverbial PM dots at that point, I knew she was much younger than I, so a loud warning bell began to sound in my head. I found myself wanting to change the subject, in case PM was contagious over the phone.

Yet I had to know the symptoms so I could (hopefully) rule it out for myself. I tried to sound casual while asking her to share some of them. I said I was asking "for someone else," of course. She cited several; night sweats being one. I congratulated myself. I had none of them. Even though I had been awakening nightly feeling *very* warm and the sheets were wet, I didn't consider that to be night sweats. There's a huge difference between "warm" and "sweating," isn't there?

# 14
## KICKING THE DOG FOOD BOWL AND OTHER TIRADES

*Next thing I knew,* my now-regular "night warms" waking me in the middle of the night began to be followed by the worst menstrual cramps I've ever had. Did I mention this was not during a period? Sleeplessness accompanied the warms and cramps. And my boobs were sore. I became more irritable.

And I'm talking irritable about *really* insignificant things like the dog food bowl being in my way in the kitchen. One evening I kicked it hard across the kitchen, right in front of my husband and son. I mean HARD! And that's a slight understatement, if you ask my husband. Eventually, a week of severe 4:00 a.m. cramps got my attention. This was followed by 45 days without a period, which was followed by a period that lasted 21 days. This finally caused me to seek medical attention. I had hit bottom.

> Dear God,
> What is happening to me? I am not myself. I feel so out of control. I want the old me back. I cannot live like this anymore. Please guide me to solutions.

PART II

# Coming to Terms

# 15

## The Doctor

*After having experienced* about four months of progressively worsening erratic physical symptoms and behavior, I decided to see a doctor. My current OB/Gyn had coincidentally retired just prior to my appointment, so I was reassigned by my HMO to a completely new doctor. She walked into the exam room and extended her hand to introduce herself. As I took her hand to shake it, I burst into tears, which continued for the duration of my visit. Again, weird-face-making crying to a stranger was not my usual style. Yet I didn't even care; I just let it happen. I loved that she patted my leg as we spoke. Six tissues later, she asked if I had ever considered meds to help balance out the hormones. Me? Perimenopausal? Definitely NOT me! I still plan to have one more baby. No, this can't be the onset of menopause. God, aren't You making a mistake here? I'm only 45!

> Dear God,
> Please guide me in this unfamiliar situation.
> Please steer me toward a solution.

# 16

## MEDS – WHO, ME ... DEPRESSED?

*When my new OB/Gyn asked* if I'd ever considered meds to deal with my hormone imbalance, I said "no." Let me interject that I will use the umbrella of "meds" here without reference to specific types of them. I have no medical credentials or medical background (except in my own mind). This is my opinion only, based on my own life experiences.

Anyway, I went home and thought about her suggestion. I vaguely remembered some caveat about the fact that the suggested drugs could have sexual side effects, and that it could take as long as eight weeks to take effect. Meanwhile, I wondered what Tom Cruise would think of me, given his recent outspoken comments about Brooke Shields' public disclosure about medication usage. It was 2005 at the time and I said: *Go, Brooke!*

These hesitations were short-lived. I couldn't stand how I'd been feeling and behaving. I was willing to try the meds. After a complete exam revealing nothing medically wrong with me, I began taking a low dose of antidepressants. I knew I could stop if I had an adverse reaction to them. Besides, the girl who did my brows at the time swore they would make my appetite diminish. A girl has her priorities, after all.

> Dear God,
> What is Your will for me? I am on the fence about drugs. Please guide me. I am starting them, so if I'm misreading You, please make Your will abundantly clear.

# 17

## Take Surveys and Ask God for Help

*Within a week of having begun the meds,* I was barely able to have an orgasm. The physical sensation was considerably less than I was used to. Here was yet another thing about me that had changed. I immediately launched my own personal phone survey among my girlfriends. As I've mentioned, I do this for everything from toenail fungus to chin hairs to how-to-do-a-playdate to what type of underwear won't ride up.

> Dear God,
> I am confused about meds. Are they for me? I know I have judged others who take them. Help me put aside my existing judgments and the judgments of others (especially Tom Cruise), to hear what Your will is for me. And could you please hurry? I may lose my mind soon if something doesn't give. Thy will be done.

# 18

## MEDICATIONS AND SEX DRIVE

*My friend Cordelia* (41) agreed with my brow babe that meds could affect sex drive. She said she eventually opted to go off meds because she was newly divorced and was having the best sex of her life with her new beau, except for the fact that it was orgasm-free sex. She happily reported her body returned to its former sensual responsiveness within one week of having gone off the meds. My brow babe, on the other hand, calmly assured me things would eventually right themselves. I just needed to ride it out, so to speak. It seemed like an eternity, but four weeks later, the esthetician's words rang true and are still doing so regularly. Thank heavens!

> Dear God,
> Please give me knowledge of Your will for me and the patience to wait till I receive it.

# 19
## Basketball Stomach Paranoia

*Evidently as we age,* it takes less "fuel" to keep our bodies running. If we don't cut back on fuel, the excess fuel consumed is stored in our bodies as fat. If a body's storage site is the midsection, the waistline can appear a little like a … well, a basketball (henceforth referred to as *the* Basketball).

Now, let me begin by saying I don't care who has the Basketball. I just don't want my body to have it. Here is my take on the Basketball. You know that waistline expansion that some postmenopausal women complain of and countless others fear? Well, I am more than a little paranoid about getting this label myself. So of course, I've done a survey among friends. Some seem perplexed as to where the Basketball comes from. My friend Cordelia (58) was determined to avoid IT. In fact, in the early years of PM, she was quite certain she had completely arrested menopause through daily soy consumption, increased water intake, regular exercise and nutritional food choices. She was into natural solutions, which worked for her for a few years. Eventually, her symptoms of feminine dryness and other PMS-like symptoms influenced her decision to use hormone replacement therapy.

Although I'm relatively new to all this, I still have my opinions. Whether they'll hold true for me remains to be seen. But I have been maintaining a 35-lb. weight loss since early adulthood through moderate eating, NOT dieting, and a daily personal connection with a power greater than myself. So that counts for something. But given my personal history, I am concerned with what my waistline will look like as I progress through menopause.

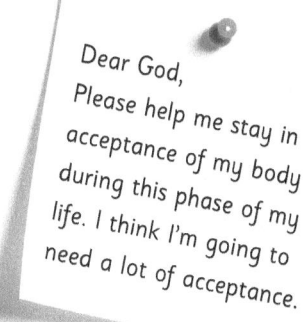

Dear God,
Please help me stay in acceptance of my body during this phase of my life. I think I'm going to need a lot of acceptance.

# 20
## "Padding" My Food

*I learned in my mid-twenties* that when I have the faith, courage, and willingness to walk through life with healthy, normal, and appropriate behavior in all my relationships to the best of my ability, I do not need excess food to cope with life. One of my favorite mentors, Raffi, always said, "Remember, Precious Angel, overweight is faulty problem solving!" I agree.

When I don't have enough faith, courage, or willingness to use healthy communication and self-care skills, I overeat. I call this temporary lack of faith, "padding my food." Padding my food means I consume just slightly (or a lot) more food than my body needs to function properly. I say temporary because if I have stayed committed to exploring each isolated bout of padding my food, I have always returned to sane eating within 48 hours or less. I suppose if I were to pad my food enough times in a row without taking action to get back into the solution, the result would be weight gain. By the grace of God, I have never had to go there in the past 30+ years. One day at a time, I have always had the willingness to look at my feelings and learn an improved, more functional method to problem-solve in any given situation. And just an FYI, padding my food has never turned out to be the solution.

Dear God,

Please give me the willingness to stop and look at my feelings and actions before I resort to padding my food today. And if for whatever reason I find myself already having padded my food, please give me the willingness to explore my feelings on paper and heal from the experience.

# 21
## A Word About Orgasms

Dear God,

How do I write about orgasms when my parents might read this? This subject is sensitive, yet so vital to my well-being. How shall I approach it? Please advise. When I was in my 20s, a wise woman friend suggested I read *For Yourself* by Lonnie Barbach. That book explains the female anatomy, including labeled diagrams of female sexual organs, describing their functions. This was not something my mother or anyone else had ever gone over with me. That "talk" they gave us in fifth grade hadn't covered this, either. The whole book is basically about how to achieve orgasm and about giving people permission to enjoy orgasms. My mother never went over this with me, either!

What great news this was for me. Additionally, the book addresses masturbation. As you can imagine, this topic was also not in any of my "mother-daughter" talks. I went on to read another book by Sondra Ray, called *I Deserve Love*. This book gave even more permission for sexual/sensual pleasure and expression using positive affirmations, no matter what that looks like for someone.

Basically, through these two books, I learned that not only is it okay for me to feel pleasure, it is vital to my well-being. Even if it means making weird faces! Having an orgasm is a way for one to get out of her head and into her body/feelings/heart, if ever there was one. And if ever my husband and I are out of sync, there's always the vibrator.

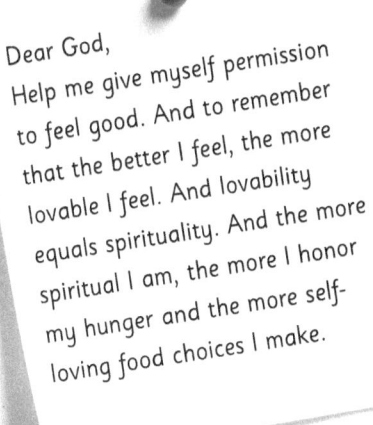

Dear God,
Help me give myself permission to feel good. And to remember that the better I feel, the more lovable I feel. And lovability equals spirituality. And the more spiritual I am, the more I honor my hunger and the more self-loving food choices I make.

# 22

## Husband Doesn't Get It

*It's a good thing I have a lot of girlfriends* because my husband simply doesn't get this whole experience and he doesn't even pretend to. He is a hardworking husband and father, for whom I have great respect. But he is not female, let's face it. Maybe you have one of those sensitive husbands. Not I. I tried to explain to him all I have been going through. Not only does he offer no solution, he offers no sympathy. Dead end.

> Dear God,
> Help me have realistic expectations. Help me remember where to turn for comfort ... and where not to turn.

# 23

## ACNE, WRINKLES, AND RAISING A PRESCHOOLER;
### the Bermuda Triangle of Womanhood

*As an adolescent,* I experienced mild acne ... nothing horrible. My skin was not the best in the school, but not the worst. I considered myself lucky. I escaped the teen years relatively unscathed as far as acne.

Okay, fast-forward to now. I am 45 years old. As I type, I have a monster undergrounder on my forehead and another huge one on my chin that just came above ground. How can this be?

Then there are the wrinkles. Sure, there are options. Dermabrasion, eye lifts, face lifts, neck lifts, breast lifts. I'm pretty gun-shy on all the above, apart from breast lifts (see "Breast Lift Reject") and dermabrasion that I still plan to try (I'll keep you posted). But lately, I consider trying things that will bring back my youth. Often.

Then there is my darling preschooler, soon-to-be kindergartner. Today, while talking to a friend of mine at the gym, I described him as a salmon flopping around me while I waited in line at the frozen yogurt store. He circled me repeatedly, touching me as many places on my legs as possible as he revolved around me. I don't have to tell you that he is taking his life in his hands if he behaves this way on certain days of the month. This is why parent-educator Sandy McDaniel coined the term "flat teeth day." Enough said.

The point is, as a woman who had her first child at 40 years of age, I am in a tough situation here and I know I am not alone. Experiencing perimenopausal acne and wrinkles while raising a preschooler is truly the Bermuda Triangle of Womanhood. Some days can be incredibly hard. Add in some sleep deprivation and night warms, and there's no telling where it will take you. This is where that idea about starting a MMOMMS Club, the Menopausal Moms Offering Menopausal Moms Support Club, would come into play, big-time.

> Dear God,
>
> Please calm me down. Please inspire me with ideas for creative outlets. Help me to see beyond what seems to be insurmountable in this moment.

# 24
# MOTY Club and MOTY Club Summits

*My neighbor Cordelia* and I are both 40-something moms of young kids. We've noticed that motherhood involves constant guilt and insecurity. "Did I handle this or that parenting situation right?" "Should I acquiesce when my son wants me to polish his fingers with my 'Sock-it-to-me-orange' nail polish for preschool?" These ponderings can occur several times per day. To assuage the nagging feelings of self-doubt without padding our food, we have banded together to form the Mother of the Year Club (MOTY). The unspoken mission statement of MOTY is "to support each other through steadfast positive affirmation of each other as mothers doing their best in any given situation." When I leave phone messages for Cordelia, I identify myself by saying, "Hi, MOTY here." When I drive by her house, I yell, "Hey, MOTY!" We even have her husband trained to say it now. Last week he drove by my house and yelled, "What a great mom!"

Sometimes I exhibit questionable child-rearing behavior (such as losing my temper or wanting to move far away from my family immediately). Or sometimes I am just having an MDK day, relative to husband, job, or any given situation. When this happens, I call a spontaneous MOTY Club Summit. They are never preplanned and are usually held at Cordelia's house because they have the kind of backyard that could hold my son's attention for hours on end. Summits can be anywhere from ten minutes to an hour, depending on how long our kids will play together peacefully. At the typical summit, I recount my questionable parenting behavior insecurity to Cordelia. Her response will undoubtedly be "Mother of the Year." And I do the same for her. And then we laugh.

This nonjudgmental response is all that is needed to bring back perspective to any situation. We are reminded that we are human and doing the absolute best we can. And we are not alone. After that, we may break into "birth" stories, or something equally fascinating. The MOTY Club Summits are a huge source of comfort for me. I love my friend Cordelia because she's incredibly open about how she's really feeling. And we share a love for using the f-word in a really mean voice when the kids are out of earshot.

I feel completely comfortable being open with her as well. We always leave summits with a smile and renewed will to persevere as sassy women who are rocking wives and moms.

> Dear God,
> Thank You for the MOTY Club! I may not have given my permission to be entering perimenopause, but I am enjoying time with my MOTY Club friends.

# 25

## THE WITCHING HOUR

*Any woman* who has lived through motherhood knows how trying those early years can be. As a mother of a preschooler-soon-to-be-kindergartner, who also works outside the home, and endeavors to respect my beloved husband, I am consistently tired beyond comprehension. I was introduced to the term "Witching Hour" by my mom friends, but basically, I think as women, we all have our personal Witching Hour times of the day.

> Call to Action:
> Call someone in the MOTY Club or a PMSS (perimenopause support squad) member for a quick Witching Hour outreach call. Sometimes we just call each other and say, "It's the Witching Hour!" Just hearing the comforting "I know ..." on the other end of the line can sometimes do a world of good!

For me, it's the time in the afternoon when it just seems like it has got to be bedtime by now, but it's only about 4:00 p.m. My Witching Hour goes from 4:00 p.m. till my son's bedtime. It includes dinner, bath time, teeth-brushing, story time, etc. It sometimes includes crankiness, on the part of mommy, child, husband, or dogs. Whether or not you have kids, I think we all have our personal Witching Hours.

# 26

## Padding My Food During the Witching Hour

*You get the idea* ... a challenging time at best if you are hoping to avoid the Basketball. The way I determined my own personal Witching Hour(s) was by figuring out what hours of the day food calls to me. For me, that's when food really tries to seduce me into some "afternoon delight." It can be awfully hard to resist. Phone calls have saved me more than once.

> **Call to Action:**
> Call someone in MOTY Club or a PMSS member to avoid faulty problem-solving with food.

# 27
## Unstructured Sundays

*I am a person who thrives on structure.* At our house, Sundays are typically unstructured. Unstructured time tends to be quite challenging for me.

> Dear God,
> Thank You for the growth opportunities that Sundays bring me. Be with me today. Use me in a powerful way. Help me connect with You during unstructured time, instead of connecting with excess food.

# 28

# Talking to Other Women; a Disappointing First Attempt

*I attend a weekly women's group.* We talk freely about everything. It has been the single most significant source of spiritual healing in my life. But in over 20 years of attending, I don't recall anyone bringing up menopause. I do it now. Often. At first, I only got responses from women older than myself who were postmenopausal. They would say, "Oh, it's so fabulous NOT to get a period anymore." I could not relate to this way of thinking. I am still supposed to give birth to a baby sister for our five-year-old son. Aren't You reading my script, God?

These women annoyed me. I wondered, "Will those meds be kicking in soon, God? If not, I may have to get an Uzi and take some people out." They giggled as they recounted how awful perimenopause was. I thought to myself, "I may have to strangle someone tonight." Don't they realize I was not actually PM yet? They should have been saying, "Oh, but you are way too young to be PM." They didn't. No one seemed to be following my script. Couldn't they readily see I looked no older than 22?

I launched another phone survey. Other women said more of the same. That nothing was physically as it had previously been. Regular menstrual cycles became irregular. Normally cramp-free women recounted tales of being doubled over in pain. Those with light flows became those with heavy flows. Nothing was predictable. One woman told me her menstrual cycles stopped for over a year, then resumed. Worst of all, everyone I asked said this wackiness went on for years! I felt sad. I felt overwhelmed. No control for years? No patterns to chart and graph? This was way too much for a cute, yet slightly OCD (obsessive-compulsive disorder) girl like me to digest. And I haven't even gotten to "Basketball Stomach" yet.

> Dear God,
> Help me remember that I have never had any control over people, places, things, and menstrual cycles. Pat Allen, PhD, MFT, says, "The way out of a negative feeling is a positive decision followed by action." I will keep talking about menopause with other women I know. I will keep writing in my journal. God, please help me to accept and embrace this change.

# 29
## New Wave Day

*Today was my monthly New Wave Day.* I mentioned earlier I have been maintaining a 35-lb. weight-loss for over 30 years. Seventy-five percent of the time, I make self-loving, nutritional food choices in moderate amounts, similar to one of the oldest commercial weight loss programs. But one of the many ways I have maintained that weight loss is through allowing my food to be imperfect. By allowing myself a release valve, if you will. Once a month, I have what I call a "New Wave Day." I eat larger portions and I eat all the non-nutritional food I can find. It's basically a scheduled break from reality. It's also a break from thinking about being PM. The following day, I have a major food hangover and remember all too clearly why I choose not to eat that way daily, as I used to many years ago. I am only too happy to return to my more self-loving food choices. I have had monthly New Wave Days for over 30 years; ever since I lost my weight. It is not for everyone, but it works for me and I am grateful for the friend who suggested it to me years ago.

The thing is, usually I still experience just as many feelings. But I end up with a new perspective somehow. It's a good thing.

> Dear God,
> I am so sick of my husband's depression and so sick of his sloppiness and so sick of his sore ankle and knees. I am tired. Taking a spontaneous walk with Cordelia was the highlight of my day. I am learning what the balance looks like between bulldozer and doormat as a wife and mom. Thy will be done (TWBD).

# 30
# Whose Body Is This?

*We all observe* our menopause experiences differently. For some, it's a gradual awareness that evolves over time. For others, it virtually seems as if the changes have occurred overnight. My friend Cordelia (50) described her menopause experience like this:

"One morning I woke up and everything I thought I knew about my body had changed. And suddenly, it was as if I was in someone else's body altogether."

> Dear God,
> Help me be patient with myself on my journey. Please give me the ability to be open-minded as my personal hormonal transition unfolds. Help me to trust that I am right where I am supposed to be today. It would really be great if You could help me change my perspective from dread and fear to excited anticipation, joy, and exuberance about what lies ahead in my Big Amazing Life.

# 31
# "Padding" My Food vs. Honoring My Hunger

*I've always found* that if I stay in touch with the will of my God, my clothes continue to fit. And if I'm willing to sit through my feelings without eating excess food, my clothes continue to fit. But when it becomes "my way or the highway," my clothes seem to get a little tighter. When it's uncomfortable to sit still and feel my feelings and I "pad" my food, I can no longer "hear" God. My clothes seem a little snug.

That philosophy for living has worked for me all these years, including before, during, and after pregnancy. Therefore, I'm thinking there will be no Basketball season in my life, as long as I honor my hunger, stop when I'm full, practice extreme self-care, honor the wall of self-kindness, feel my feelings without padding my food to the best of my ability, and stay spiritually fit. In other words, "getting and staying thin between the ears."

Getting thin between the ears may sound like a lot, but don't worry, we're in this together. One of the reasons I wrote this book was to tell stories of how I do that: one day and one feeling and one incident at a time, with the help of God and other women in my life. Keep reading. More will be revealed.

> Dear God,
> Please help me stay in the present and stay willing to be thin between the ears.

# 32
# Unpacking "Getting Thin Between the Ears"

*On my journey toward better health,* I realized that my overweight condition was the product of two things. The first was a damaging diet mentality—or mindset—which kept me endlessly and unsuccessfully on overly restrictive diets. The second was my emotional eating. The restrictive nature of the diets I chose heightened the emotional eating cycle because portions were either too small or food variety too limited, or both. For that reason, whenever I was in the diet phase of the cycle, I was physiologically hungry to begin with. My judgment was impaired–it was a foregone conclusion that I would deviate from the diet in a big way. It was just a matter of when. The inevitable feelings of shame I experienced each time I "failed" on another diet caused me to eat even more, hence the cycle continued. It's a classic chicken-or-egg situation,

> Dear Universe,
> I know You have big plans for me. Please use me in a powerful way.

but whether the diet mentality caused the emotional eating or vice versa is immaterial. The point is, to the degree I believed "this next diet" would be the solution, I would never be able to break the endless cycle. This diet/emotional eating cycle kept me in a destructive, emotional-shame spiral for over six years.

The important thing to note is that there is a solution for both. Before I was able to let go of the accumulated excess weight on my body, I had to completely change the way I thought about, and talked about, and treated my body. I call this process of mental re-configuration "getting thin between the ears." For any personal growth to be lasting and permanent, the process of getting thin between the ears must precede it.

Once I was thin between the ears, my next step of personal growth came from increasing my emotional literacy. I realized the importance of looking at the feelings underlying my behaviors. Slowly I began the process of learning to emotionally regulate, or "feel" my feelings. Unless I improved my emotional literacy, the same feelings would continue to fester, having no outlet to be expressed.

Call to Action:
Do you believe in the Diet Mentality? What does it mean for you? Are you willing to let go of that? If not, think about how it has worked for you, if the definition of a diet "working" means losing weight and keeping it off for over a year.

# 33
# Emotional Regulation

*As I've mentioned,* my journey to better health began when I focused on getting thin between the ears, coupled with becoming emotionally literate. As I intentionally changed the way I thought about, talked about, and treated my body, I simultaneously worked on becoming emotionally literate. I learned to identify, express, and process feelings and move on. This skill is also known as emotional regulation.

According to Dr. Hillary L. McBride, who was a featured guest on Jen Hatmaker's "For the Love" podcast "Undoing the Shame of Our Body Image Struggles" in episode 3 of 2019, the research being done on mental health issues shows that most mental health issues are primarily emotional

> Dear Universe,
> Thank You in advance for the ability to change the way I think about, talk about, and treat my body. Thank You in advance for the ability to increase my emotional literacy. I am teachable.

regulation disorders. It is quite common for people not to know what to do when big emotions arise … or they are not feeling any emotions … or they don't know how to express their emotions in ways that are supportive for themselves or others.

This sounds like me. I experienced all three mentioned above. The journey to becoming emotionally literate has been years long and continues today. It has involved sitting in uncomfortable feelings—a lot. It has been awkward. It has been messy. It has had setbacks. It hasn't been perfect. It was—and is—indescribably freeing and wonderful. I am still on that journey, 35 years later. I wouldn't trade the experience for anything. Join me. You'll be glad you did.

> Call to Action:
> If there's one thing you could do to help yourself, it would be to learn how to feel feelings. Are you brave enough?

# 34
# Buzz Lightyear Birthday Party

*Throwing parties is something I dread.* I don't particularly like going to parties either, because I feel socially awkward. My son's fifth birthday was in July. I have only thrown two parties in my life. One was for my husband's fiftieth. The other was a combination first birthday for my son and fifty-something for my husband. This year, for the first time, my son asked for a birthday party. Moreover, he has been telling me his proposed plans for this party for months. My friend Cordelia (37), who is the mother of 6-year-old twin boys, informed me that I need to honor his request and that he is now too old for me to change the subject regarding his party request. I am constantly amazed that his intellectual capacity continues to increase. In any event, Cordelia urged me to walk through my fears and have a party. I agreed, on the condition that she will be available for daily party consults by phone prior to the party.

I had no sooner made my decision than the bullhorn in my head began to blare: "No one will come!" "You will have lame food!" "You will have lame games." "It will be a flop!" "How will you know what to buy?" S.H.A.M.E. = Should Have Already Mastered Everything. NOPE!

> Dear Universe,
> Please give me the courage to walk through these uncomfortable feelings. Please remind me that I don't have to do this perfectly. Please remind me that I do not have to have already mastered this.

# 35
# Drug Seems to Kick In – Husband Helps to Fill in the Blanks

*One date-night* walk with my husband, after the meds had seemingly kicked in, we talked about PM the most we ever had. As we walked, I tried to recount when my erratic behavior had begun. I had thought it was that day of sobbing to my son's preschool teacher in February. My husband gently reminded me of *several* PM behaviors he had taken notice of that predated February.....

Dear God,

Help me be brave enough to be open with another person about what I am going through. And please give me the ability to choose a safe person who will honor my process. Thank You in advance for clarity on all the above. Some sleep wouldn't hurt, either. Please and thank You.

# 36
## Read a Book on Menopause... ANYthing but That!

*My friend Cordelia* (48) is almost completely menopausal, so she's like a mentor to me. I called her today and complained about everything in my life for 15 minutes. I finally got to my feelings and began to cry. "I feel like my life is over. I'm not young anymore," I lamented. "Men will no longer look at me and I was just getting comfortable with myself and my body (these past 10 years). I am so sad about all that. I fear being considered obsolete by society. And so sad that the whole second-baby wish will be gone forever. And have I mentioned how old I feel? Did you ever feel any of this, Cordelia?" There was a short pause and a little sound came through the phone that told me she was smiling.

Cordelia is happily married and has no children; she doesn't want children. I know she can't relate to me on the baby issue. And as far as the youth/male attention issue, she replied, "Honey, that's just not true." Obviously, she knows something I don't; I could hear it in her voice.

Cordelia again suggested I read *The Wisdom of Menopause* by Christiane Northrup, MD. I fought the urge to slam down the phone and erase her number. I loathe reading books to learn about getting old. In fact, I loathe most self-help books, but especially books on menopause. Besides, I already skimmed the menopause section of Northrup's other book, *Women's Bodies, Women's Wisdom* that I had bought for my mom. That should be enough.

Okay, I'm not going to tell Cordelia, but I did order The *Wisdom of Menopause* book everyone is raving about and it arrived yesterday. But I am not going to read it —yet. I don't even want to open the shipping box. If I don't see the book, then this whole PM thing might not actually be happening. I think I'll go to lunch.

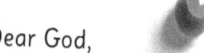

Dear God,

Please give me the humility and open-mindedness to work through my innate contempt prior to investigation and try something new and/or take a suggestion. But also help me remember that my journey is uniquely mine. It is not supposed to look like anyone else's. Just because others are ready to read Dr. Northrup's book does not mean I need to read it. Maybe I'll decide to read it some other day ... or not. My timing and choices are perfect for me.

# 37
## Picking Fights With the Massage Therapist

*Then there was the time* I got irritated with my massage therapist. I almost cried as I said, "Now I am so mad I don't even want to stay for the massage!" We talked things through, and it all turned out to be a misunderstanding, but the point is, if I am getting stressed out at a massage, there is something going on with me.

> Call to Action:
> Be willing to sit still and listen when experiencing uncomfortable feelings. Write down what you feel. Be open to something good coming from it.

# 38

## Forgetfulness: License to Interrupt at the Gym

*One day at the gym,* I knew I was starting to have a morsel of acceptance of my condition, even though I did not give my permission for my body to experience PM. One of my friends recommended a surfing video I could buy for my husband's birthday. The video had a two-word title. Surely I could remember that until I got to the car to write it down. She said it to me several times to be sure I had it. I left the gym elated, only to realize the name had escaped me already. I ran back into the gym to ask again. By that time, my friend was busily engaged in a conversation with another woman I barely knew. I completely interrupted them with my question, pleading "sorry, menopause!" The two women laughed knowingly and didn't mind my rudeness a bit. I can't believe I'm saying this, but I guess there *could* be some advantages to this ...

> Dear God,
> Please help me be patient with myself and my memory. Give me yet another dose of extreme self-acceptance about where I am today.

# 39

## This Feeling, Too, Shall Pass

*OMG!* I woke up feeling the best physically I've felt in weeks. I'm so grateful. Could it be the asparagus I ate last night? There I go, trying to discern the pattern. I love patterns. No matter, I guess. Just enjoy! Embrace the lifting of the physical blahs. Yes, feelings really do pass. Once again, God, You remind me of this. Thanks! And of course, since I feel better physically, I feel better emotionally and spiritually. Was it the writing in my journal I did last night? Or is it because it's Wednesday? Anyway, I am grateful for whatever tripped my positive feelings.

8:15 a.m.
Just after preschool drop-off. "She" talked to me . . . the younger mom! And I had the nerve to roll down my car window and initiate conversation with her, with no makeup and marginal hair, on my way to the gym. And she was nice

to me! MOTY! And she's coming with her daughter to my son's Buzz Lightyear birthday party, even though her father is probably the same age as my husband! I can do this "life" thing! I feel exhilarated!

9:30 a.m.
Lately in my exercise classes I have felt like I had lead in my shoes. I attribute this feeling to the PM experience as well. But today in my "Step Extreme" class at the gym, I felt like my old self about being light on my feet. So I'm in the ladies' room at the gym after class, feeling like an Olympic athlete, and my head goes, "You know, you'd better have decent food at your son's party for the parents or the party will suck and everyone will think you're lame." Nothing like a major endorphin buzzkill. I make a mental note to call Cordelia, who has volunteered to be my informal party consultant.

9:00 p.m.
It was a total "green light day" today. I took a risk today and took my son to a pool party. It was one of those pool parties where the planets aligned, and all the kids there got along well. And I liked the moms there—all two of them—and it didn't really matter that I was closer in age to the one grandmother attending than I was to the other moms.

On the way home, we dropped by my soul-mate mom and neighbor MOTY's house, just in time for leftover pizza. She is my age and I can speak without editing a single word I say. What a gift. And she has this fabulous backyard that my son will play independently in for several hours.

> Dear God,
> Just thank You. Tons of gratitude for these great feelings while they last.

# 40
## Green Light Days

*You know when you are driving someplace* and every light turns green just as you approach? Even the lights that usually stay red super-long are all green. Well, when this happens, usually everything else also seems to go well that day. It's the strangest thing. My son is easygoing and doesn't try to torture the dogs. My hormones cooperate with my agenda. I feel on top of the world. I only have a green light day about once every three months, but they are magnificent!

> Dear God,
> Thanks for this green light day. I really needed it. And thanks for the best night's sleep I've had in weeks, also. The reprieve from "night warms" last night was appreciated

# 41

## Glasses for Reading (working up to it for two years — baby steps)

*I have had perfect vision my entire life.* I have always been the only one in my family who doesn't need to wear glasses, until three years ago. When my son was a baby, it became increasingly difficult to decipher the dosages on his Baby Tylenol bottle. I finally realized it was my eyes that were the problem, and not a cruel extra-small print trick that Tylenol was playing on tired moms. It was determined at an eye exam that I needed glasses just for reading. I chose some glasses reluctantly and promptly put them in an attractive faux leopard case, never to be removed. It wasn't that I was opposed to wearing glasses, necessarily. I just could never remember to put them on. I had glasses for an entire year, but the glasses rarely left the case.

At the eye exam the following year, it was determined that I needed a slight correction for both near- and far-sightedness. Again, I complied and got another more stylish pair of glasses that I proceeded *not* to wear. This time it was recommended I get progressive lenses, which I learned are a more high-tech version of bi- or trifocals. They suggested I try wearing progressive sunglasses, since I was having such a hard time accepting myself as a glasses person. I could do that. I wear sunglasses all the time. First time I wore my new prescription sunglasses I wasn't yet used to them and walked straight into a low tree branch that left a mark between my eyes. Just another reason for me to feel old, clumsy, and ugly. It took me quite a while to make peace with glasses. This whole glasses thing was a terrible blow to me. I take everything as a competition—it's just my personality. I had always thought I was just a little superior to the bespectacled population. There went that thought.

On the third year's eye exam, a slightly stronger reading prescription was needed in my progressives. I chose frames for the third time in my life. My husband hated them. I had then decided to have the rejected pair made into glasses that transition into sunglasses and took my husband back to the shop with me to select frames. He has a good sense of style and color. We found something we agreed upon. I'd say I wear some pair of corrective glasses 75 percent of the time now. But my point is that it has taken me three years to get to this level of acceptance of them. I have been gentle with myself. Wearing glasses ties into the whole aging thing. Now that I am PM, I am much more sensitive about aging. Did I just declare that I am PM? Oh, sorry, that must be a typo. Now that I may be PM, I am much more sensitive about aging.

> Call to Action:
> Practice extreme self-gentleness as it relates to your self-talk, even if it takes you three years to embrace a new idea. Think of a similar situation where you could possibly be gentler with your self-talk and not let the barking-dog voice enter.

# 42
## Breast Lift Reject

*I kept talking about PM* in my women's group and with all my friends. I quickly found that many women had no interest in the subject, and I didn't blame them. Either they were too young to relate, or they were in denial and thought as I had, that if they didn't discuss it, it would go away. But this made me feel separate from many of my good friends. My own mom had had a hysterectomy, so I couldn't really talk to her, either. I felt sad about the whole thing and uncertain of myself. Was my life over? I was often tired from the night warms that left me unable to go back to sleep. I noticed I frequently lost my train of thought mid-sentence. I made more mistakes. I forgot things. I recently drove away from my home without my purse twice in one week. And I am not the forgetful type. All these things made me feel old for the first time. For some reason, I became convinced that a breast lift would solve all of this.

Prior to breastfeeding my son, I was a 34D. My boobs have always been pendulous, but I liked them just fine. Post-breastfeeding, I am a 36C, but I am uncomfortable with the way my breasts hang. It is almost impossible to find bras that fit comfortably, look feminine, and make me feel normal looking in clothes. I went in for a $50 consultation with a surgeon who turned me down. This was yet another reminder that self-esteem is an inside job. To this day, I am thankful for that surgeon, because he knew that changing my outside appearance would not be the end-all to my body image struggles. And his honest advice saved me $9,000!

> Dear God,
> Help me to remember You love me and my entire body as it is so much. And that what I look like physically has little to do with my worth as a spiritual being on earth.

# 43
## Getting Dressed for the Gym

*Talk about being sensitive about aging*—getting dressed for the gym in the morning can be stress-inducing. Can I wear this outfit? Will others look at me and think, "Oh, someone needs to tell her she's too old to wear that." Does the "V" in my workout top line up with my cleavage?

And if I do decide to go ahead with the chosen outfit, hoisting my boobs into my workout top is a whole other story. I don't know what happened after nursing that glorious baby of mine, but my pendulous breasts became pendulous-squared. And even then, my bras must be equipped with global positioning capabilities to be sure the pendulous situation is kept in check. There's a lot of bending over and hoisting activity when I put on a bra. And that's just phase one. Phase two is nipple location. I wish someone would make a nipple-leveling tool. The whole breast/nipple longitude-latitude issue is more prevalent at the gym than in street clothes. The point is: PM exacerbates so many situations. Or is it the other way around?

> Dear Universe,
> Please help me accept my entire body as beautiful the way it is today. In accepting myself as I am, I accept Your will.

# 44
## Victoria's Secret Bras

*I mentioned earlier* that after having a child, it was almost impossible to find bras that would fit comfortably, look feminine, and make me feel normal-looking in clothes. I finally accepted myself as I was, and don't you know… They invented a new bra! When I first saw the commercials for these bras, I snorted, "OMG, they make it sound like it will change your entire life or something! How ridiculous. It's *only* a bra!" Not that I have anything against Victoria's Secret (VS), of course. It just seemed like hyperbole.

A few weeks later, I happened to be in VS looking for PJs. As I was escorted into the dressing room by the head Bra-Meister (as I called her from then on), she casually asked if I would like to try on the new model I'd seen advertised. I said, "Sure, what the hell." Well (insert angel music sound bite here), I am here to say that commercial is completely accurate. The bra provides the most lightweight, comfortable, sassy, and perfect boob location I have ever experienced. And they come in tons of different colors. I have swapped out all my bras for these in every color I can get! I went home and practically started a phone chain to let all my friends know the good news. We are all wearing them now. Thank you, Bra-Meister, wherever you are!

> Call to Action:
> Maybe it's time to be refitted by your favorite Bra-Meister. Permission granted!

# 45
## Acid Reflux Acceptance
## (How-late-in-the-day-can-I-eat-chocolate-without-it-affecting-my-sleep-that-night?)

*I have Acid Reflux,* aka GERD - Gastroesophageal Reflux Disease. I have had the diagnosis for about three years, but I probably had it way before that and didn't know it. Thank goodness for my ENT doctor (ear/nose/throat) for connecting the dots. I had chronic post-nasal drip; nausea before, during, and after eating; heartburn in the middle of the night; nightly coughing attacks at 3:00 a.m. that left me in tears holding the wall for balance; and chronic colds that literally lasted for weeks.

My darling husband built a special wooden wedge to elevate the head of our bed four inches. I take medication. I have altered my diet to discontinue eating after 6:00 p.m. Imperfectly, I admit. I was told to reduce consumption of alcohol, caffeine, mint, and chocolate. I have not had an alcoholic beverage in over 30 years, nor had caffeinated coffee more than one time every six months, and mints are not really my thing. I have always had my chocolate-chip cookie day once a week and my monthly New Wave Day usually includes some form of chocolate, but I would hardly call that excessive chocolate. Yet, I still have this disorder.

It took me months to be in acceptance about having it. Don't I have enough on my plate, God? But the miracle is, my appetite has decreased noticeably, and food just doesn't give me the high it once did, for the most part. So, I have realized that can work in my favor, relative to the Basketball stomach. And through talking about it openly, I have learned some great pointers, one of which is that if I consume the chocolate item before noon, I can usually still get a good night's sleep. As usual when it comes to food, I have discovered a way around feeling deprived. That's why I always recommend taking surveys on everything!

Dear Universe,
Here I am again, asking for help on acceptance of something about myself. But I know You love this and all my quirks and are only too happy to help if I am willing to stop beating myself up. Deal.

# 46
## MENOPAUSE MATH:
## Hormone Fluctuation + Existing Physical Conditions > Sum of Its Parts

*I have experienced foot issues.* Without completely boring you, I have experienced a condition called plantar fasciitis which is quite painful at times. Although I have researched and tried many possible solutions (physical therapy, acupuncture, sports massage, the MELT Method, exercise, no exercise, orthotics, ibuprofen, rolling the arch of my foot over a frozen water bottle, rolling the arch of my foot over a golf ball, to name a few), the pain persisted on and off for years.

To complicate matters, I also have misplaced fat pads on the soles of my feet, resulting in no cushion when my feet hit the floor. In short, if my bare feet meet the floor for more than about two minutes, it hurts. Even slippers are uncomfortable, unless they have custom arch supports in them. I am not telling you my foot saga to get pity from you, but rather to point out that we all have our Achilles heel (or sole or arch) in life to deal with. And dealing with these various conditions during PM can contribute to my crabbiness.

> Dear Universe,
> Help me never to give up on finding solutions to whatever I am going through. Please bring me new ideas and open-mindedness. Thank You in advance.

# 47

## PERIOD BEGINS,
### but I am sure this time it's just pregnancy spotting and not my period.

How cute am I?

> Call to Action:
> Today might be a good day to take a nap.

# 48
## Chin Hairs – Baby Steps

*The facial hairs* draw my forefinger to them. So annoying. Negative self-talk in my head. Repeat. I need to break this cycle. But actually contacting the electrolysis place seems like too much effort. Time for baby steps. Just locate the electrolysis number for now, and then I will call tomorrow. Sometimes baby steps are all I can handle.

Call to Action:
Is there something you've wanted to do, but can't quite bring yourself to do it? How about making a positive decision followed by action? For today ... just look up the number and write it down some place. That's enough for today. Tomorrow is a new day.

# 49
## Migraines: 6 Cordelias

*One symptom of PM* that I have so far escaped is migraines. At least six of my friends report suffering from migraines, relative to their menstrual cycles. Further, three of those six no longer have periods, yet still have the migraines. I will keep you posted throughout the year as to whether I get one. But for now, as with every other PM symptom, I give us all permission to research self-loving solutions, whatever that may look like.

> Call to Action:
> Research self-loving solutions on your own timetable.

# 50
## Sad About PM

*Today I feel sad* and overwhelmed about transitioning hormones and all that signifies to me.

> Dear God,
> I feel sad and overwhelmed. What will this new normal look like? Please give me the willingness and the ability to sit with the feelings without padding my food. Please send comfort in some nonedible, nonshoppable, nondrinkable form.

# 51

# HOME ORGANIZATION PROJECT
## The "Denise-ification" of Our Home: Part I

*Our home has clutter.* Every home I have lived in as an adult has had it. I don't know how not to have it. I have a December wedding anniversary and birthday. Last December, I told my husband I could make his Christmas, wedding anniversary, and birthday shopping easier for him. I requested a visit from Denise, an image consultant. He readily agreed since he hates shopping and never knows what to get me.

Denise came to our home and together we reviewed every piece of clothing in my closet. When she was finished, I was left with approximately a third of my clothes. It was way overdue! The next day, we went shopping to bring the inventory back up. I now have a closet stocked with color- and garment-coded clothes that mix and match, complete with jewelry and shoes. It's been quite an experience. Because Denise is so skilled, I spent way less money than expected, including paying her hourly shopping rate. It was worth every penny.

But it didn't stop there. Next, we addressed my son's toys. *Before* Denise, my son's toys inhabited literally every area of the house ... *every* area. I think it took a while for me to grasp that this being I gave birth to at 40 years old was going to be staying with us for a long time, so I needed to make room for him. *After* Denise, my son had places for all his belongings and Denise showed him where everything went so *he* could maintain order right along with me.

We weren't done! The office was ready to be tackled. By that time, there was no stopping. We continued to the kitchen, guest room, the laundry room, and all closets. We even set up a gift-wrapping area in one closet. As we progressed over the months, it became readily apparent that I would not be finished until I had conquered the ultimate ... the garage. Having an organized garage is something I have barely dared even to dream of. Yet as the months of working on the house went by, I began to see light at the end of the tunnel. The garage was completed within five months of having begun Project Denise-ification.

The home organization project has truly been a spiritual experience for our family.

- ✓ It has improved my relationship with my husband.
- ✓ It has improved my parenting skills.
- ✓ It has improved my self-confidence.
- ✓ It has improved my peace of mind.
- ✓ It is satisfying to live in my organized home every day.

Denise-ification was a gigantic undertaking and during the months-long process, many uncomfortable feelings came up. Oh, it was expensive. There were tears and there were fights, but in the end, it was all worth it. There are no words to describe the freedom this experience has brought me.

> Dear Higher Power,
> Help me be willing to try things that are way out of my comfort zone. And if something is Your will, please bring me resources who can help me with the process.

# 52

## Home Organization Project
## The "Denise-ification" of Our Home: Part II

*As I've mentioned,* the home organization project was truly a spiritual experience for our family. It improved my relationship with my husband. It improved my parenting skills. It improved my self-confidence. It improved my self-esteem. It was continually satisfying to be in my home.

But at the time of completion, my friends were dubious. Would I be able to maintain it? It has been years since Denise's initial visit and most of my clothes are still in order. I almost always hang up my clothes immediately when I take them off. It's a great feeling.

Having never lived clutter-free, one thing I hadn't anticipated was that you must work to keep things in order, especially when you live with two other people. Part of this journey has been learning how much time to allocate to keeping things in place per week. So far, it seems to be taking about one hour per week.

The other shock was that, although my husband loves the new look, and it was his idea (brought up in marriage counseling as his #1 complaint about me!), he does not participate in upkeep. Thankfully (and after major attitude adjustment on my part), I know where everything is (even in the garage), so my son and I handle the upkeep, for the most part. I guess he figures that he worked to pay for most of the work Denise and I did, and that should be enough on his end. I can sort of see his logic if he agrees to have a hardscape and landscape design drawn up for the yard. But that's another story. And after all, I did get the plantation shutters I have wanted for my entire adult life. The money I make teaching group fitness classes doesn't quite cover that.

> Dear God,
>
> Please give me the willingness to explore ways to keep my nervous system as balanced as possible. What will my part look like? What are realistic expectations for time and money?

PART III

# Embracing

# 53
## Who Am I? What Is the New Normal?

*I feel like myself again* for the first time in two months. Maybe the whole PM thing was all just a dream and it's not really happening. I feel so "back to normal." I am sure I will stay feeling like this for the rest of my life, right? In fact, I am so sure that there is no need to continue writing this book. Well, okay, I'll keep writing, but just to help my fellow Varsity sisters who still suffer from what I used to have.

My husband and I actually had sex today! Yes, on a weekday. Yes, in the morning. Yes, before our preschooler awoke. Wow, we're on fire.

OMG, a cute young guy said hello to me at the

> Dear God,
> Just THANK YOU for today. As my friend Cordelia (35) would say, this has been a "Pretty Woman" day! I am incredibly grateful to have had a day where I feel like myself again.

gym today. One of "the regulars" has allowed me into the Inner Circle of Gymness. I am euphoric. Strangers are smiling at me in Costco, and vice versa. All is right in my world. And I'm not even perspiring.

# 54
## Witching Hour Tales

My son and I arrived home about 6:00 p.m. from the day's activities and I was starving. My Witching Hour is generally between 4:00 p.m. and 8:00 p.m. Even though my PM "crazy" meter was only on moderate-to-low today, my son started to get on my nerves. He told me I wasn't his friend because I no longer allow one of his unruly playmates to come into our home. Crying followed. All I wanted to do was eat dinner! Costco granola began calling my name from the kitchen. How did it know my name? I went to it. We had a "quickie" and I came to my senses. I took a deep breath. I got out the

> Dear Sally-Girl,
> Great job with your food choices and portion sizes for today. They were exactly right. I love you no matter what you eat, and I love you no matter what you weigh. You are doing the absolute best you can, and I am so proud of you.
> Love, Big Love

veggies. It's funny how veggies never know my name. Nevertheless, I was somehow able to find them. My food choices weren't perfect, but I could've eaten way more. Nothing tastes as good as self-loving food choices feel, especially when I wake up the next morning.

> Call to Action:
> Write yourself a letter of encouragement, telling yourself what a great job you did on something. It can be from your wise inner self, your compassionate parent, God, or anyone you feel safe with and loved by.

# 55
## Still Got It

*Another guy* in the Inner Circle of Gymness said good morning to me today! Maybe I am not over the hill just yet.

> Dear Higher Power,
> Help me to realize I am not obsolete. I am not invisible. I have value. Of course, men will still notice me. What's not to love? My life is SO not over. I still have a lot of living to do. Thank You.

# 56

## VPLs and Unstructured Time

*This morning* as I chose what to wear, I was uncharacteristically obsessed with not having visible panty lines (VPL). It took three different pairs of underwear before I was satisfied I could leave the house.

I haven't opened THE book yet. I've procrastinated three weeks at this point. Weekends are not a good time to be reading about menopause because lots of feelings come up for me on the weekends. During the work week, my time is structured, with driving my son to school, and then driving myself to work, etc. Weekdays, it's easier for me to choose self-loving amounts of nutritional food. But weekends are another story. They bring unstructured time, down time.

Feelings come up for me during down time. In my women's group yesterday, I felt sad about the baby thing. I really don't want my childbearing years to be over. It seems too soon. I let the sadness come. I cried again. I didn't pad my food. If I padded my food, then I'd still feel sad AND I'd have a stomachache. Then I'd be irritable to my family, whom I love dearly. I feel grateful for having the willingness to experience the feelings without spontaneously eating.

Unstructured time on weekends also means time with two other people with two other agendas. And yes, the two people are the husband and child I have hoped for since I was 12. And as strange as it may sound, it is challenging for me to be with the two most important people in my life for two days in a row without structure! Thankfully, on this Saturday I've got a kid's birthday party to go to with my son.

And I thought it was all about VPLs today. Also, my boobs hurt today, nothing major, but enough to notice.

> Dear God,
> Give me balance today as I spend intimate time with my family. Help me discern the difference between control and healthy self-care with boundaries. I don't want to be a bulldozer or a doormat. How about something in between?

# 57
## Surfing – My Antidrug

*You may remember* those public service ads that used to air on TV where people spoke about their personal way to fight drug abuse? They'd say things like, "Tennis is my antidrug." Well, I've decided I need a "PM antidrug" to combat going crazy during PM. I need something to take my mind off PM. Something to take the PM edge off, but in a constructive way. I have decided I will learn to surf. My husband has surfed on weekends for 35 years. Our five-year-old loves the beach and shares his dad's love of the ocean. After eight years of being a "surf widow," it occurred to me he's probably going to surf forever. So, if I am going to be spending all this time at the beach, at least I could get some exercise by surfing while I am there.

The words "I am ready to surf" were barely out of my mouth and we were in the surf shop getting all the stuff. I was nervous. What if I don't stick with it? This means I'll be a newcomer. I HATE not knowing how to do something. And having people watch. Yuck! But when it became 51-percent uncomfortable to sit on the beach another minute, I was willing to walk through my fears.

I surfed for the first time on Sunday, July 10, 2005. As soon as I was in the water, all the fear of what people would think of me vanished. It was obvious I was new at it and I didn't care! I was exhausted in 30 minutes. I stood up once or twice … barely. I came out of the water with my legs feeling like wet noodles, but jubilant, nonetheless. Surfing was my new antidrug. It's something to challenge my body and spirit the way writing challenges my mind and spirit. Fantastic!

Taking up surfing has many side benefits I hadn't even considered. My husband is ecstatic. It brings our family closer together. He and I have different hobbies. Surfing was something we can all do together that's relatively inexpensive. I love wearing a full wetsuit—I don't have to spend so much time applying sunscreen. I get a break from being a mom. It's just with God, the waves and me. My husband loves teaching me and being the expert. I get to respect him for his mind and physical strength.

> Dear God,
>
> Help me continue to find ways to stimulate my Body/Mind/Spirit that doesn't involve spontaneous eating, even if just for this one day. Thank You.

# 58

## Beach Day and Living Life

*Off to the beach* for another family beach day and surfing. No time to write now. Living life.

9:00 p.m.
I really wanted to eat beyond the point of being comfortably full tonight, but I didn't. I feel so content right now. So then why did I want to eat spontaneously? Sometimes I think I am even uncomfortable feeling content. I am surfing again tomorrow and feel so proud of myself. I've decided to set a goal of catching two waves each time I go into the water with the option of catching more.

> Dear Big Love,
> Please help me remember to take You to the beach with me and give me the ability to honor my hunger. Also, please give me the ability to sit with uncomfortable feelings, no matter what they are. I deserve contentment.

# 59

## Legal Appointment Fears: Taking Baby Steps

*Today my head's telling me* I need to call a financial planner to get our affairs in order. I read enough of Suze Orman's *Nine Steps to Financial Freedom* to know we need to set up a revocable living trust, and then promptly cast the book aside. My husband and I have chosen our son's legal guardians, but have never made it legal. I've gotten names of financial planners from four good friends, but still haven't called one. Why? Because that negative voice in my head says, "What will you say when they pick up the phone? You will sound ignorant. You may stutter. You are 45 years of age and can't even formulate an intelligent sentence on this topic. OMG! You might as well go eat a big brownie instead." And so it has gone for months.

I often encounter this type of negative banter in my head. Fear of the unknown. Fear of sounding stupid. Fear of pretty much everything. I've found I just need to break things into small increments. Remember, I'm the one who hasn't opened the shipping box that contains the menopause book. But at least I have moved it near my desk now.

Anyway, for today, I commit to get the phone number of one financial planner. Not to *call* it. Just to write it down. This is my self-loving contract for today. I know how much I love myself by the contracts I'm willing to make and keep as Dr. Pat reminds me. A self-loving contract per day keeps the Basketball at bay.

And by the way, my boobs hurt.

> Call to Action:
> Is there some action you've wanted to take but it just seems too hard? How could you break it down into smaller increments to make it seem less daunting? ... gentle, gentle.

# 60

## Wacky Gratitude List

These days I'm constantly checking in with myself, leery of the sequel to *Hormones Gone Asunder!* After all, I reason, I've had like three rational days in a row. That's about all I get per cycle these days. Granted, my boobs seem to hurt throughout the entire cycle, but I'll take what I can get. It's as if someone authorized simultaneous nipple piercings for me, without my knowledge. Then there's the issue of constantly feeling warm. Is it hot in here?

Author Melody Beattie says, "Gratitude leads to acceptance." When I think God's getting His plan all wrong for me, I write what I call a "wacky" gratitude list.

- I'm grateful my boobs hurt.
- I'm grateful I'm going through PM even though I never gave my permission.
- I'm grateful I've only got one child.

- I'm grateful my husband is cranky tonight because he just found out he needs foot surgery.
- I'm grateful I have a respectable husband who cherishes my feelings 51 percent of the time.*
- I'm grateful for my loving, precious son.*
- I'm grateful I did not kick the dog food bowl across the kitchen today.*
- I'm grateful I must wear glasses now to read.
- I'm grateful I've made nutritional food choices in self-loving amounts today.*

*P.S. It's okay if some real gratitude accidentally creeps into the list.*

> Call to Action:
> If you think God's getting His plan for you all wrong today, write your own wacky gratitude list and see what happens.

# 61

## Journal Writing to Avoid the Basketball

*My husband* watched a show called "Nanny 911" on TV with me last night. I love this man! Today I'm having minor intermittent cramps. Could I be pregnant? I got the elliptical trainer that is positioned directly under the ceiling fan at the gym today! I don't ask for much in life.

My son's fifth birthday is in less than two weeks. In many areas in life, I'm confident. I'm confident about my ability to eat in balance, for example. In areas where I haven't much experience, however, I'm not confident. Having birthday parties for young kids falls in the latter category. But I'm walking through it. RSVPs are arriving on our voicemail. I am uncomfortable because the messages aren't giving me a head count so I must call people back. I'm discovering when you have kids in school, it means talking to parents you don't know. That's scary for me. And now I must bother them twice! You may think this sounds crazy, but for me, walking through life's daily minutia can take me to the fridge before you can say, "thick frosting on carrot cake." So that's why I am committed to consistently writing, to access my ongoing daily fears, minimize the negative self-talk in my head, and discuss and plan for whatever action I am afraid to take.

> Dear Sally-Girl,
> I know these calls are hard for you. And I know you will make them anyway. If only you could see yourself the way these other moms do. Who is this kind voice calling me? Just like the way I see you. I'm always so happy to hear from you.
> Love, Big Love

# 62

## Throw Money on a Feeling

*I don't like feeling feelings.* I know it's important to my well-being to feel them. So, I do. But not without first trying a few alternatives to avoid them. One alternative I gravitate toward is spontaneous eating, to stuff feelings down. Another technique is to throw money on a feeling. Tonight, I bought workout shoes online. Okay, no big deal, I work in the field of fitness, right? And they also happened to be 25 percent off. I bought four pairs! At times when I suspect I may be throwing money on a feeling, I do a letter-writing exercise that goes something like this:

*Dear Sally,*
*If your personal workout shoe inventory was totally adequate as is, and you weren't obsessing about it, what would you be free to feel?*
*Love, God*

*Dear God,*

*I feel worried about Mom. She's chronically ill. I'm anxious about my husband's medical consultation tomorrow for his ankle surgery. How much extra work will it be for ME post-surgery? And how successfully will I handle taking care of him? How will my son's birthday party turn out? Will I be able to sleep tonight? I'm approaching the hormonal-maelstrom portion of my menstrual cycle. What will this month be like?*
*Love, Sally*

Now I read what I have penned and notice that basically all these worries are about things I can't control.

Dear God,
Please comfort me tonight. Help me remember to give these worries to You. And to trust Your plan as each moment of my life reveals itself. Help me to let each moment unfold.

# 63
## MDK Letters

*As I have mentioned,* a willingness to identify and feel my feelings is not my default. Part of the reason I dislike feeling them is because you cannot schedule them. I love my schedules and routines! Another reason I dislike them is sometimes they feel super big and as if they will never stop. And some of them are strong, dark, and negative. If people knew how strong, dark, and negative some of my feelings are, they might not love me anymore. Yet I am committed to living my fullest life with the full spectrum of feelings, whatever they may be.

One of the ways that I stay committed to living my fullest imperfect life is to make up names for some of my feelings. It comforts me and makes me smile. It reminds me that I am human and doing the best I can. Whenever I feel super mad about something, I call it "Murder-Death-Kill" (aka MDK), a phrase I discovered in the sci-fi action film

*Demolition Man* with Sylvester Stallone, Wesley Snipes, and Sandra Bullock.

There is a writing exercise I do when I am having MDK feelings and thoughts. These are feelings and thoughts I would NEVER act on—you know what I'm saying? Basically, I write an MDK letter to the person/place/thing/event. The recipient of the letter will NEVER see this letter. It is for me only. This exercise enables me to feel all the feelings and move beyond them.

> Dear God,
> Remind me it is safe for me to identify and feel the full spectrum of my feelings and to trust that I can learn how to do this in a healthy, normal, and appropriate way, without excess food, and without hurting anyone. Teach me how to do this with writing tools and to be an example of that to my son.

# 64
## Is It Hot in Here?

**Call to Action:**
A. Write a letter to your version of a higher power, telling him/her how you feel. **Realistic Goal:** One sentence, with the option to write more.

B. Have your version of a loving higher power write a response to your letter. Ground Rules for letter B:
1. Addresses the concerns expressed in first letter A.
2. Make it longer than first letter.
3. Make it consist of only positive responses. If you can't think of anything positive to say, just write the opposite of what is said in the first letter, even if you don't believe it right now.

*It's only 8:00 a.m. and I am warm and already irritated. I'm in that "get away from me" mood again.*

*Dear Big Love,*
*I feel irritated because I am warm already and it makes me feel old, unattractive, and obsolete. Love, Sally*

*Dear Sally-Girl,*
*I love you so much I can't take My eyes off you. I'm sorry you are uncomfortable due to the heat, but please remember I have so much in store for you today. Please keep your eyes open.*
*Love, Big Love*

# 65

## Mini Naps

*I was going to write in here,* but I decided to take a mini nap first …

I'm back. The nap was five minutes max. Sometimes I just need to get horizontal with eyes closed for one minute with the option to do longer and it makes all the difference.

My husband had a consultation regarding a proposed surgery on his foot. I got dressed up and asked if I could go along. The only time we've ever gone to doctor appointments together was when I had my amnio when I was pregnant, so this was a big deal. I even skipped my Cardio Dance Party class at the gym. It felt good to go and just be there with him. I resisted the urge to sign him in, offer to fill out his paperwork, or speak for him in the presence of his doctor.

I reminded myself I wasn't there to be his mother; I was there to be his partner. I kept my mouth shut, even though I am incredibly knowledgeable about practically everything.

It felt wonderful. I made self-loving food choices for lunch as a result.

I feel so tired. I may open the shipping box that came from the bookstore (weeks ago) tomorrow. Today I kept busy with my to-do list all day. Sometimes I am a "human doing" to avoid feelings. I forget I am a human being. If I slow down, I will inevitably feel feelings. I know it's not logical, but I'm afraid I may die from feelings.

Dear God,
I feel sad about going through menopause. I don't want to age. I don't want to grow old. What will I be like? Will I still be sassy and cute? I really wanted to have another baby. I love having a child, even though parenting is way harder than I ever imagined it would be.

God, I also feel close to my husband lately. Like we are getting still closer. My decision to learn to surf is somehow related to all this. I don't know. I get these intuitive ideas that I believe to be from You, God. When I get these ideas, I listen and act. When I make self-loving food choices, these ideas come to me more readily. When I choose non-nutritional foods and large portions, I am blocked from receiving these ideas. God, please help me with self-loving food choices and appropriate portions today. I am worth it!

# 66

## Critical Voice/Compassionate Voice: Part 1

*At the risk of sounding completely crazy,* I have a lot of voices in my head on any given day. I like to think it is because I am an intelligent, creative person. Whatever the reason, a lot of these voices say critical things to me—a lot of the time. It's unpleasant. I call this Negative Self-Talk (NST). Sometimes before I am even able to identify that NST is going on, my best thinking tells me I should eat Cheez-Its or some other non-nutritional food right now. Or that I should eat an exceptionally large portion of food. In the past, overeating was my go-to solution to quiet negative self-talk. From about age 12-24, this was pretty much my standard coping mechanism. From age 18-24, it became so common for me that I gained weight. For that six-year period, I was consumed in a continual binge-eating/dieting/fasting/over-exercising/body-distorted/self-loathing/perfectionistic cycle.

Through a series of self-care actions including self-help groups, therapy, and a fierce commitment to find a solution, I have lost the excess weight and have maintained a perfectly imperfect healthy lifestyle ever since. I have a daily reprieve from that cycle if I stay in fit spiritual condition. Those critical voices still talk in my head at times. When they do, sometimes I respond by eating excess food. But sooner or later, I use a tool to get into the solution and quiet them.

One tool that works especially well for me I call Critical Voice/Compassionate Voice (CV/CV). In this exercise I write two letters: one from that "Critical Voice" (my dark side) to me and one from what I call my "Compassionate Voice" (my bright, positive side) to me. As with many of the writing exercises I do, I typically read it to a person I trust when I finish. A wise friend once told me, "Writing is putting it in the garbage disposal. Reading the writing is flipping on the disposal switch." In other words, in reading my written thoughts aloud to God, myself, and another human being, the healing goes to a deeper level and I love myself just a little bit more.

The rules of this writing exercise are that the second letter must always be written at the same sitting as the first letter, and it must be of equal length or longer. And the purpose of the second letter is to counter the negative statements in the first letter with self-loving statements.

*My Critical Voice:*
*Dear Sally,*
*This entire book idea is so lame. What are you thinking? How pompous of you to think your ideas are of interest to anyone! And just the editing of the book will be way too much work, let alone getting it published. Do you know how hard it is to get published? And you were so stupid to tell all your friends, because now someone will beat you to the punch and you will just be wasting your time.*

*My Compassionate Voice bubbles up:*
*Dear Sally-Girl,*
*I am so proud of you for listening to that still, small voice within. What a wonderful experience for you to write this all down. Remember, when you're in God's will, all expenses are paid. If it's God's will, it'll work out. As far as editing goes, take one day at a time. The goal's not really to get published anyway. It's the process that's so healing for you. Embrace it as you already have. It's okay. Don't worry about who you've told. You're just so excited. And you've such conviction about your vision. Go with it.*

Always remember, God loves you so much He can't take His eyes off you!

# 67
## Is This My New Normal?

*I'm feeling cute today.* Maybe I still have a modicum of pulchritude in me. The cabinet guy even told me I looked good yesterday. My husband couldn't sleep at 3:00 a.m. and, of course, neither could I, so we channeled that sleeplessness into a good thing. Thank goodness our son's a sound sleeper!

> Dear God,
> Please give me the willingness to suit up and show up for life today and to keep an open mind about how things "should" go today. Thank You.

# 68
## CRAMPS

*I've been having bad cramps* since this afternoon. On top of that, my feet hurt. It's two weeks before I would normally get my period. What's going on? I hate this. I think I'll go have some frozen yogurt and go to bed.

> Dear God,
> When I am feeling low like this, the question is always the same: Do I want to live anyway? So far, the answer has always been yes.

# 69
## Embracing Cramps

*I am wakened by severe cramps* at 5:00 a.m. I can't go back to sleep. Tears are close to the surface. I don't want to be going through PM. These are those same cramps I had three months ago and haven't had since … until now. Author Melody Beattie says, "Gratitude Leads to Acceptance."

I rolled over in bed to snuggle with my husband but he's not there. I get up to find him, and just as I suspected, he is lying in bed with our son, talking. Mostly, it's our son who's talking, as usual. Every so often, our son will listen as his dad sings parts of songs and our son will sing back to him. Then he continues "reading" books to his dad. I secretly sit just outside the door and listen to this tender father-son moment. The moment I might have missed if I hadn't been wakened by cramps. Thanks, God. Gratitude leads to acceptance.

Dear God,
I am grateful to be having cramps.
I am grateful my husband and son have special times together.
I am grateful I can't predict what my body will do from one moment to the next.
I am grateful I appear to be PM.

# 70

## Lower Expectations to Below Sea Level

*It's my husband's birthday.* I'm obsessed with the chocolate cake I've ordered for him. How great it's going to taste. Then I remember people come before food! I'm spending the day with my husband; our son's at preschool today. Staying present with my loved ones is intimate. Intimacy does not come naturally to me. It's safer for me to obsess about the cake. It's going to have some type of incredible

> Dear God,
> Help me to remember my worth is not contingent upon another person's mood. Remind me my husband has every right to his feelings. Help me to remember that today is more about relationships with people than about relationships with food. It's about letting people be themselves and loving them anyway, myself included. Even if we are both down.

chocolate filling, after all. I keep spotting pregnant women today. Some days are like that. I feel sad I'm not one of them. It's supposed to be me, but I'm having menstrual cramps without a period instead. But I digress. Gratitude leads to acceptance ….

My husband is always depressed on his birthday. I labor over his gifts in hopes of cheering him up. It almost never works. Today is no different. I feel disappointed. Hence, I obsess on cake.

# 71
## THE CAKE

*Well, the chocolate cake* was beyond my expectations because it had thick frosting. I like a little cake with my frosting. But it was so good I decided not to honor my hunger and kept right on eating. Some days are just like that. One day of overeating does not make a Basketball stomach. It's just a signal to me that I'm trying to avoid feelings about something.

My feeling today was of frustration with my husband. Why can't he be more upbeat on his birthday? It would have been nice if he gushed over the thoughtful gifts I gave him, as I would have had it been me.

I eventually realized by day's end that my husband's mood has very little to do with me. He's nervous about his upcoming foot surgery. I further am reminded that I'm not lovable just because of my "performance" relative to his birthday. I am always lovable. My husband adores me and I him.

As an exercise to get in touch with how I feel, I write letters to people that I plan NEVER to give them. I talked about this earlier in my journal, but it bears repeating. My letters don't have to be polite or grammatically correct and usually, the more swearing the better! If I were to do this exercise today, it would have been directed at my husband! Then I read them to a safe person without revealing the "intended recipient." It also feels good to read the letters in a dramatic voice. I heal on a deeper level because my subconscious mind thinks I really said these feelings to the person. Writing is like putting my feelings in the garbage disposal; and reading my writing (in this exercise, it's a letter to nowhere) is like flipping the switch. I really like this analogy because it creates a very visual picture.

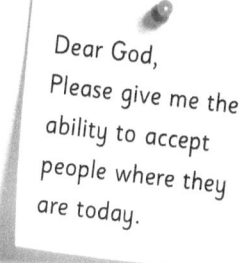

Dear God,
Please give me the ability to accept people where they are today.

# 72
## THE MAELSTROM

*I am quite sure* the hormonal maelstrom is in full force for this cycle. It was windy at the beach today and the flapping noise made by the umbrella almost caused me to be homicidal. Finally, it was so bad I asked my husband if we could leave the beach. I feel restless. I can't relax. There are a few less flies alive in our home now. The fly swatting was cathartic for me. My boobs hurt.

> *Dear Big Love,*
> *I feel sad about how all these random things bug the hell out of me. Like wind. Like fans. Like flies.*
> *Love, Sally*

> *Dear Sally-Girl,*
> *I know, Sweetie Pie. I know this is hard. Hang in there. This, too, shall pass. I love you so much.*
> *Love, Big Love*

# 73
# Drinking Water

*We all know drinking water is important.* There are scientific reasons to drink water. It helps maintain the balance of body fluids, which are important for digestion, absorption, and maintenance of body temperature, among other things. Hydrated skin looks better than dehydrated. Your kidneys work better at ridding your body of toxins. Adequate hydration prevents constipation.

> Dear Universe,
> Help me have the willingness to take precious care of my body. What a miracle it is to see how it functions.

# 74
## BUYING SOME TIME BY DRINKING WATER

*We know there are scientific facts* about why drinking water is good for us. But there is also a spiritual component to water consumption. I am by nature an anxious person. Pretty much everything causes me to be anxious. And food is readily available in most situations. If you are prone to using food as comfort, this is an unfortunate combination. Situations where I perceive I am expected to be perfect—like meeting new people, or anything new—cause me to be nervous. Situations I cannot control make me uneasy, as well as any kind of transitioning. Sometimes, all of those collide simultaneously. For example, whenever I go out to eat, it's a transition from being alone to being with another person. To calm myself down, I use the spiritual component of drinking water. I order a glass of water as soon as possible and drink the entire glass right away.

> Call to Action:
> If you tend to feel anxious, try drinking a glass of water as soon as you encounter the feeling.

# 75

## Yelling Is Not a Spiritual Solution

*My boobs hurt;* I have cramps. I'm too hot and it's only 8:00 a.m. I feel nauseous. My son kept pushing me to get a stuffed animal for him and I just snapped. I yelled, "NOOOOOOO!" as loud as I possibly could and went out into the garage. I felt immediate shame for my behavior. The shaming voice in my head proclaims, "You are fat, and you are ugly. No one likes you AND you are a bad mother, wife, human, pet owner." Within a period of five minutes, I have apologized to my family. But the shaming voice continues relentlessly. I went to my women's group, feeling terrible. While there, I had a moment of clarity.

I realized that I could tell my son (and husband) that I am working on this inappropriate behavior. The shame I experienced comes from my forgetting that I am not expected to be perfect. With this awareness comes immediate release of shame. What a relief. What a great model for my son as well. Perfectionism takes on so many forms for me. I am constantly reminded that as a recovering perfectionist, I need only strive for mediocrity.

> *Dear Big Love,*
> *Thank You for putting angels on this planet who teach me how to live.*
> *Love, Sally*

> *Dear Sally-Girl,*
> *I am here. I will never tire of telling you your shame is optional and that I love you not only in spite of your imperfections, I love you because of them.*
> *As always, Big Love*

# 76
# NEW WAVE DAY

*Yesterday was my New Wave Day.* It's my scheduled monthly break where I choose to eat larger portions and non-nutritional food. And now, as usual, my stomach hurts. I am so tired. This day seems overwhelming. My husband is a saint because he occupied our son so I could sleep till 9:30 a.m. Still I don't think I can stand this day. I fear it will never end. It's only 10:00 a.m.! My son is perpetual-motion-personified as he jumps from one agenda to the next. "Mom, can I touch your breast?" "Dad, what does heaven look like? Can we go kayaking today?" I managed to get myself to the shower.

I ask God for a solution. It comes to me…. I ask my husband to watch our son so I can go to the gym. This is hard for me. I feel depressed and hopeless. I make the bed. My son is panting like a dog as I write this.

> Dear God,
> Please help me to get through this day. Thank You for helping me to think of a solution. I feel depressed and hopeless. Thank You for inspiring me to make the bed. I keep reminding myself: baby steps.

# 77
## SUNDAYS ARE THE WORST

*Today is Sunday.* After much deliberation, we ended up going surfing together as a family. I am proud of myself for surfing again today.

Now I am so tired, but it helped me feel a lot better after calling my friend Cordelia simply to complain and swear. Being a mom is hard. And I only have one child. I hate to admit this, but the Universe knew what she was doing when she only granted me my son. Being a wife is equally hard. The degree of difficulty of both combined is exponentially greater than individually. I'm not sure why, but when the three of us are together as a family unit, I find it especially stressful. I continue to question why that is.

As much as I'd like to eat my way through my Sunday discomfort, I know excess food would only intensify and prolong the discomfort. Yes, Sundays are the worst.

Dear Universe,
There is nothing like cold sheets on a summer night after a day of self-loving food choices. Thank You. Goodnight.

# 78
## Flopping Like a Salmon

*What I want to say to my son right now:* Stop talking; Stop wiggling. You are so annoying me! Stop flopping around like a salmon. Stop making repetitive sounds in the dog's face. Stop being five!

Sometimes I need an attitude adjustment. When I find myself talking like that, I know it's one of those times. When I am the parent responsible for my child, solutions for my anxiety are a little more limited because I cannot just abandon him and go for a drive. Here are a few actions I take to get out of a nasty mood:

Ask God for help

Go into the bathroom

Go Out Doors … my friend Cordelia taught me this one … it can be seen as an acronym for GOD.

Brush my teeth

Put on music

Sing

Put on music *and* sing

Make a wacky gratitude list

Call someone on PMSS (perimenopausal syndrome squad)

> **Call to Action:**
> List three options you can use to change your attitude.

# 79
## NEGATIVE SELF-TALK: PART 1

*Here's what my head's saying:* "Just eat that last piece of cake. Your son's party will suck on Friday."

I don't even want to write in my journal today because I don't want to deal with reality. I keep saying, You don't need to be writing a book about PM. Besides, no PM women want to hear about you being all whipped up or verklempt; overcome with emotion about a birthday party." But that's where I am today.

*My Critical Voice:*
*Dear Sally,*
*Just eat the cake. You weigh too much, and your food is all over the place. You will gain all your weight back. Your son's party is going to be a flop. No one wants to hear what you have to say. No one cares how you feel or what you think. You have no value whatsoever.*

*My Compassionate Voice:*
*Dear Sally-Girl,*
*Your son's party will turn out just the way it needs to be. The only important thing is that your son enjoys himself. I love you whether you eat the cake or not. I know you are sad today about being perimenopausal when your plan was to have more children. I have really great things planned for you. Please keep your eyes open so that you don't miss them.*

Always remember, God loves you so much He can't take His eyes off you!

# 80

## NEGATIVE SELF-TALK: PART II

*Here's what my head's saying*: "What are you thinking? You can't write a book. Don't even bother writing today."

The novelty of book-writing has worn off. I love my husband and son today. It's as if yesterday's feelings never happened. Good thing I didn't act on them, although I did have that last piece of cake.

I chose self-loving foods and amounts today. I enjoyed the smell of the freshly laundered washcloth as I washed my face at the end of the day. When I don't pad my food, I enjoy things like that. My boobs and lower back hurt. As my period obviously approaches, I feel sad that the end of my childbearing years is eminent. A girl at the gym returned today for the first time since having delivered her second child. I forced myself to congratulate her on her new arrival. I hope my face looked normal when she told me, "It's a girl!"

*My Critical Voice:*
*Sally,*
*Don't write this book. What a waste of time.*

*My Compassionate Voice:*
*Dear Sally-Girl,*
*If you weren't so busy berating yourself, what would you be free to feel?*

Always remember, God loves you so much He can't take His eyes off you!

*Dear God,*
*This hurts. Ever since I can remember, I have dreamed of having children, plural. It's really starting to look like that's not Your plan. Why not? I feel sad. I feel angry. Thy will be done. You suck.*
*Sally*

*Dear Sally,*
*I know sometimes it is hard for you to accept My plan as it unfolds. It's okay for you to feel sad. And I can certainly handle your anger. And I love your blind faith in My plan. Trust the plan. You're gonna love it, I promise.*
*Love, God*

# 81

## Party Countdown

*I am freaking out* about this upcoming birthday party Friday for my son. The guest list is up to 25 kids and 35 adults. I am holding it in a park that I'm not even sure I'm allowed to use. I had to have extra party favors overnighted due to my compulsive over-inviting issues. This is why I don't throw parties! That critical voice in my head goes on overdrive! Will people readily discern I am the mother, not the grandmother? I don't really care that much about that. But will I be sweating like a rock star and therefore have bad hair? Now *that* is what I care about.

I decided to call four people on the PMSS and feel much better. Just hearing that I am not alone is so comforting to me. Breathe!

> Call to Action:
> Is there an upcoming situation in your life that you're anxious about? Think about how you could reframe the way you think about it so that you can enjoy it.

I am reminded by one PMSS member that this is about *fun* … and my son. I'm given a reality check. It's not about my hair being perfect. Oh, yeah! Thanks.

# 82

## Day Before Party

*I feel horrible physically today.* I'm nauseous, hot, almost like I'm going to throw up, but not quite. I don't want to write because I don't want anyone to know I get like this. I feel depressed … hopeless. I am sad to be PM. Worn out from magnified premenstrual symptoms for the past two weeks, but today was the worst yet.

My son was so annoying and needy today while we got ready for school. I held onto an ice cube to diffuse my impatience with him. I did not yell, although it took everything I had. I went to the gym, and then called three women on the PMSS.

It was the first time I'd tried the ice cube trick. I always rationalized that "I'm not mad enough to waste an ice cube, and I don't want my hand to get wet." When I was really mad, I promised I would try it. As if there would be some sort of criminal offense for excessive ice cube usage. So today I finally had to trick myself into trying it by saying, "It's okay to waste this ice cube. And it's okay to try this even if it seems really stupid."

After all this obsessing about the party, I noticed a small rash on my son's chest this morning. I immediately future-tripped to what a hassle it will be to call the 60 party guests tomorrow to cancel because he has scarlet fever. I decide to call the doctor and make an appointment for him instead of keeping my radio tuned to "KF***." I refill my mega water cup with ice and drink.

> For today, I will keep my radio tuned to "KJOY" rather than "KF***" by taking action. I will use my intellect to make a positive decision and follow by acting on that decision.

# 83
## Party Day

*I can't sleep.* My throat is scratchy. I have a continual stream of party details marching through my head. At this point I am more excited than nervous, but both feelings seem the same physically: an upset stomach and the inability to sleep coupled with exhaustion. I drank a vitamin C drink with a honey chaser. I am so excited to have taken a risk and asked people for help with the party. What an enormous relief. And now I wonder if I have enough blankets for the kids to sit on at the party?

On the PM front, I am noticing at this time of my cycle—the three-plus weeks of magnified premenstrual symptoms—that my appetite is diminished. The amounts of food that I usually consume seem like too much. I want to remember to honor that, rather than go on autopilot while eating, so I can honor my hunger and not pad my food. By "padding" my food, I mean consuming just slightly more food than my body needs to function properly in any given situation. Also, I am constantly warm lately and it is annoying. I carry a huge insulated frozen water bottle around constantly. The feeling that I could use a shower is ongoing and irritating.

I keep forgetting to talk about my forgetfulness and inability to focus lately. It is increasingly frustrating to me. Being the adorable, obsessive-compulsive girl I am, I have never been one to misplace things. However, I have left the house two times without my purse this month and yesterday I wandered around the house for ten minutes trying to find my purse … same thing with my keys.

Gratitude leads to acceptance:
- I am grateful I can't seem to keep my train of thought.
- I am grateful for my forgetfulness.
- I am grateful I have a scratchy throat.
- I am grateful I am exhausted at 4:00 a.m. yet can't sleep.
- I am grateful for PMS.
- I am grateful I will be taking my son to the doctor today, the day of his party.

- I am grateful I had menstrual cramps for the 3rd day in a row at 3:00 a.m.
- I am grateful I have had to urinate 5 times in the last 2 hours.
- I am grateful the light bulb above my head keeps flickering as it threatens to burn out.

Dear God,

Please give me the ability to be present for the party. To remember the point: be with my fellow man/woman/child. How my hair and outfit look is secondary (albeit a close second). Sometimes I get it reversed. Thy will be done.

# 84
## After the Party

*If sweaty squirt-gun-soaked kids* and adults running around for two hours straight is any indication, the party was fabulous. Everyone told me how much fun they had. *I* even had fun. I am so proud of myself for throwing it. I can't get over how much help I received from four good friends. I am just so amazed that people would help me like that. I am so touched. I hope I can sleep soon because I'm officially wiped out.

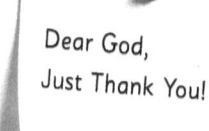

Dear God,
Just Thank You!

# 85

## Walking Through Fear

*All day today* I've been both so proud of myself for throwing a party and so incredibly drained. The PM combined with exhaustion make it hard to complete sentences today. I feel like I'm losing my mind … really.

I have a fear of throwing parties. This is only the third party I've given in my life. That's how scary it is for me. What if no one comes? What if everyone comes and it's boring? How does one know how to synchronize the endless details? Where does one draw the line on who to invite? How much is it all going to cost? Pondering things like this usually causes me to forget the whole idea in nothing flat. But a while back, my good friend urged me to honor my son's request to have a party for his birthday. I acquiesced on the condition that she would help me with details.

My son ran wild in a huge park with his friends for four hours straight. It was a massive success. But the success entailed so much more than that for me. It was quite an effort to make a list of everything I'd like help with. And it took a great amount of nerve to ask friends to help me. It was extremely touching as four women showed up early to help with the party. And, as with the two other parties I've given in my life, I was shocked that people showed up! There were sixty adults and children, to be exact. And then I enjoyed myself and it appeared the guests did as well. I hardly saw my son the entire party and was told by another mom that this meant he was having a good time.

I took on a fear and faced it head on. I feel exhilarated. I kept saying to my guests, "Hey, this really IS a party, isn't it?" I just couldn't believe I did it. Sometimes the things I am most afraid to do turn out to be the most fulfilling. I am so glad I walked through it.

> Dear God,
> Thank You for giving me the courage to walk through fear. I'm so glad I did!

# 86

## Conflicting Expectations

*Sundays are the worst.* Unstructured time with my family and we have conflicting agendas. I want to clean up all remnants of Friday's party and/or sleep. My son wants to be attached to my side around the clock. My husband wants us all to go to the beach, but he's in too much pain from his ankle injury to go surfing.

Nevertheless, he tried to blame the fact that he's not at the beach this beautiful day on me. I'm expecting spouse and child to be showering me with praise for the spectacular party I just gave. I'm still tired, but better than I was yesterday.

I feel overwhelmed with work that needs to be done on the house. It's literally never-ending. Perfectionists don't do well with "never-ending." But I've spent the last eight months organizing the house, and I'll be damned if I'm going to let it lapse back to what it used to look like. Can you imagine what the day after a party would look like around our home before the Denise-ification?

> **Call to Action:**
> This is a self-care challenge. Unplug for 10 minutes with the option to go longer. Now lie down for one minute, with the option for longer. Eyes closed. Head on a pillow with another pillow propped under your knees. Give yourself bonus points for shoes off.

# 87

## Basketball Preoccupation

*I am preoccupied* with the Basketball right now. I have been since around 4:00 p.m. today, ever since I put on this certain pair of jeans. I padded my food at dinner tonight. I kept eating after my body said it'd had enough. What am I trying to avoid feeling by over-eating and being Basketball-obsessed?

> Dear God,
> Help me remember it's not about the Basketball.

I'm still high from the party experience, yet I feel a little lonely. I have the husband and child I've always wanted. So why is this? My husband's freaking out about his upcoming ankle surgery and preoccupied with setting up our TV in the new cabinet we had built for it. This is not about me. Learning to be flexible with another human being under the same roof on Sunday is one of my greatest challenges in life. I've made it through yet another Sunday without blemishing my husband by criticizing or harshly judging him. I'll do my nails and go to bed.

# 88

## New Normal?

*I have so many conflicting feelings* right now that I want to scream as loudly as possible. I feel so crazy, my head's about to explode. It took everything I had not to scream at my son while getting him ready for school. His only "crime" was wiggling like a five-year-old. The desire to get away from him and be alone was intense. And then the guilt feelings for feeling that way are equally disturbing and uncomfortable to me. And just as all this was flying around in my head, a pregnant woman walked by me in the gym. I walked out of the gym and went back to my car to take a deep breath. It's that strong. I'm going back in now. I know the exercise will help me ride this out without taking inappropriate action toward myself or others.

Dear God,
Please give me strength to carry out Your will for me today.
Give me the faith to wait before reaching for food to stop these feelings. Just for one minute.

10:10 a.m. – Post-workout
Feeling better. But lately, multitasking is becoming a thing of the past. Come to think of it, single-tasking isn't going too well either.

4:00 p.m.
Today everything seems like the absolute end of the world. Although I would never act on it, I fantasized about taking a baseball bat and breaking a huge glass bottle display in the grocery store. I know logically it's not that bad, but my brain is saying so many negative things in my head and I can't get it to shut off. The solution is to ride this day out without excess food, and call someone on the PMSS. Faith.

9:00 p.m.
I chose self-loving food choices and amounts today. I feel so uncomfortable and I'd rather eat, but the kitchen is closed till tomorrow.

Call to Action:
If you feel like Cheez-Its are the answer right now, what would happen if you paused, asked the Universe for help, and waited for a few minutes?

# 89
# CRITICAL VOICE/COMPASSIONATE VOICE: PART II

*My Critical Voice:*
*Sally, you were so stupid to go to the lake for so long with Cordelia and her kids today. You really should have those party thank-you letters out by now. And you were disrespectful and a freak to your husband yesterday for wanting to clean up from the party instead of going to the beach with him and your son on a beautiful, sunny day. You are getting the Basketball. You're a bad wife and a bad mom. You're so sweaty and gross all the time now. And you mixed up who gave which gift to your son. And you shouldn't have let your son see all his gifts tonight. The house is a huge mess and everything Denise did is all undone now. And you'll have to have huge, uncomfortable battles with your husband about getting rid of that ugly TV stand, now that the new cabinet is finished. And the yard will always look like white trash. How dare*

*you want to spend money on the yard when you aren't even working full-time. You were a bad hostess because you were so whipped up and verklempt—overcome with emotion—at the party.*

*My Compassionate Voice:*
*Dear Sally-Girl,*
*You went to the lake for a break and to be with Cordelia. It's okay in your excitement that you forgot you hate sand and heat and lake water, and especially all three combined. And how smart of you to at least take your own car and leave when you did. The thank-you letters can wait. You have worked your butt off on the house for over eight months and love how it looks now. You have your home organized the way you have dreamed of for your entire life. Of course, you'd be concerned about getting things put back in their places as soon as possible. Especially considering the clutter you lived in for so many years prior to this. And besides, your husband couldn't have gone to the beach because he's in too much pain. He just wanted someone else to blame.*

*You are about to get your period. You always feel bloated at this time of the month, even when you don't pad your food. Way to go, by the way. Taking the veggies to the lake and all the water you've been drinking is what I call "Extreme Self-Care." I love that! And it's so okay that you got a break from your son after all that time together and work you did. It lets you treat him in a loving way when you pick him up after this break.*

*I know this sweating and being hot thing is hard for you. It seems never-ending and I know it makes you feel unattractive and unfeminine. But it will end, and you are quite feminine. And it's so normal that you got a little confused on the gift opening. It was a zoo! And this is the first birthday party you've had to deal with, really (where your son is old enough to "get it"). You wouldn't ever be expected to do it perfectly, and especially not on the first time. It's all okay.*

*It was an amazing party. You did GREAT! Everyone had fun. You lived life. You got out there and did it. Way to go! I am so excited and proud of you. You will find a place for all the toys. It's all going to work out. And your husband will find something to do with the TV stand. I know you are super-worried he'll put it in the garage for years. It's okay that you want a beautiful home and yard. Keep asking for what you want. It's okay that you aren't working full-time outside the home right now. You are raising your son. And I love you madly. Your food is fine, your weight is fine. You were a warm, outgoing hostess who hugged each guest and kept the party on track.*

*Always remember, God loves you so much He can't take His eyes off you!*

# 90
## Murder/Death/Kill (MDK)

*Today was one of those days* where I needed some attitude adjustment. Writing an MDK letter was just what I needed to shift my critical mindset to one of compassion.

Husband: your procrastinating is making me crazy! Quit leaving half-finished projects around the house! I'm sick of seeing screwdrivers, ladders, tables, wires, wrappers, socks, shoes, hangers, and popsicle sticks everywhere I turn. Next thing you know you'll want to park a car on the lawn.

Writing MDK letters helps me identify my feelings. Once I identify and express my feelings in a healthy, normal, and appropriate way, I am able to discern what action, if any, I need to take next.

> Dear God,
> Please help me come from a place of compassion for all people in my life today. Help me to determine where I need to set healthy boundaries. And please give me the courage actually to set them.

# 91
## CRITICAL VOICE/ COMPASSIONATE VOICE: PART III

*I woke up with cramps,* but the 22-year-old at my son's preschool asked me how I stay so thin. What cramps? Funny how I can give an external comment so much power.

10:47 a.m. OMG, Ellen DeGeneres showed up at my gym and did our warm-up with us in Cardio Dance Party class. Her camera crew filmed the whole thing. I am so star-struck right now. What PM? But I was sweating behind my knees today and it bugged me.

> *10:17 p.m. My Critical Voice:*
> *Sally—you are such a bad parent. You're unable to stay in the present. All you do is rush him through whatever the activity is (getting ready for school, dinner, going to bed), without ever stopping to enjoy things ... always*

*on task. How mean, cold, harsh, abusive. Even with the thank-you notes for his birthday. Even with assembly of his gifts. And on top of that, you have him in full-time preschool. He must feel so unloved. How horrible.*

*My Compassionate Voice:*
*Dear Sally-Girl ... I love you, no matter what. You are one of the most conscientious parents there are. You are being way too hard on yourself. Staying in the present is extremely hard. Everyone struggles with that. You are expecting way too much from yourself. I know this is all so new for you still. It's a process. You are so involved in your son's life. You are also kind, warm, loving, and consistent. Everyone's got a dark side and no one's perfect. I know you are doing the best you can. You are raising him with manners. He feels so loved by you for many reasons you haven't even considered. You have no perspective at this moment. It's okay that you have him in full-time preschool. As an only child, he learns vital social skills in a loving environment*

> Call to Action:
> Spend five minutes talking to someone important in your life in person. Make eye contact. Read one page of a spiritual book with the option to read more.

*that doesn't exist at home with no siblings. You are teaching him discipline and self-care by enforcing consistent bedtimes. And you've given him an hour window this summer and have been flexible with your husband's late homecomings from work. And you're just doing your best.*

*Always remember, God loves you so much He can't take His eyes off you!*

> Dear God,
> Please help me enjoy each moment more, and to give my son and husband more eye contact. Thy will be done (TWBD).

# 92
## Shave Legs, Wash Hair, Put on Makeup Day

*Today I know my period's coming* any time now. I found myself not wanting to shave my legs or shower and not wanting to wear makeup. Instead, I did all three, against my better judgment. I also chose self-loving foods and amounts, exercised, made eye contact with both my husband and son and asked God to help me stay in the moment with my family. I also apologized to my husband for being disrespectful the other day when I told him to stop eating crackers and chips after 7:00 p.m. Even though I know I am correct, it's not my business to educate him on things like that. I want to be his wife, not his mother.

My boobs only hurt a small amount today. Maybe it was the tofu in my smoothie?

Call to Action:
Pat Allen, PhD, says, "I know how much I love myself by the contracts I'm willing to make and keep." What self-care contract are you willing to make and keep today?

# 93
## Period Starts

*I feel nauseous.* I had trouble sleeping last night. I went to the gym for self-care, regardless. As I pulled out of the gym, donuts came to mind as a solution to the nausea and fatigue. I'd already had breakfast. I chose not to act on the donut idea right now and decided to review that idea again at lunch.

12:30 p.m.
No wonder I was nauseous. I got my period after about 2-3 weeks of premenstrual symptoms. Now the wave of sadness is washing over me, but also relief that I still get my period at all. I will never completely give up my second baby dream till my periods have been gone for at least a year. TWBD.

I drank a big glass of ice water. I unloaded the dishwasher and reloaded it with the already-accumulated dirty dishes in the sink.

Dear God,

Please be with me as I embrace this sadness. Please comfort me. I called someone in the MOTY club. Every feeling has a beginning, middle, and an end. I'm so proud of myself for making self-loving food choices today, despite a strong urge to stuff down my sadness with food. It took a lot of faith that I would live through these feelings without excess food. Tomorrow's a new day. My boobs hurt. God, please help me sleep soundly tonight, without interruption.

# 94
## SADNESS & LOSS

*I am the designated leader* at my women's meeting today. How can I share something inspirational when I feel such sadness and loss right now?

Call to Action:
Suit up and show up. You need to be willing to walk through uncomfortable feelings to get to the other side. Write down an uncomfortable feeling you struggle with and then write down underneath that feeling how you plan to address it for a positive outcome.

Dear God,
Please speak through me today at the meeting. I feel sad about the eminent end of baby possibilities.

# 95

## SUPER NEEDY DAYS

*I feel super needy and lonely today.* I have one free hour right now while my parents are babysitting my son, and no one can meet me for lunch. I might perish. I'm dying. I'm going to have my favorite self-loving salad at Daphne's Greek Café, even if I'm a party of one.

On my way home, my friend Cordelia called me back. Maybe it was because of the four messages I left her this morning. I toured my neighborhood in my air-conditioned car while chatting, gathering enough energy to go home and face the weekend with all the unstructured time weekends bring. And all the communication that is required. This weekend is a bit unique. My sister-in-law has offered to have my son spend the night—Saturday night. I struggle with this, but force myself to put my husband first and spend time alone with him. I'm taking a nap right now. It's so hot outside. Lately it seems like I'm perpetually "glowing" from head to toe. I'm preoccupied with whether my brand of antiperspirant is working or not.

It's 6:15 p.m. and I just had a big argument with my husband. We yelled. I guess this time alone is scary for both of us. I have been sitting alone in the kitchen doing nothing for five minutes. I literally don't know what to do with myself. What is the next indicated step? I am kind of paralyzed. After we had words, he left the room. I don't know where we are at this moment. Is dinner still on? I say the serenity prayer. So far, this intimate time together doesn't feel good at all. I can't seem to distinguish between a legitimate gripe with my husband and PM issues at this moment.

Finally, the prayer kicked in and I made a positive decision and unloaded the dishwasher, rather than my initial decision to eat a bagel within reach of where I was sitting. Then I decided to fold some laundry, since the appropriate words to say to my husband hadn't come to me yet. He came back downstairs to the room I was in and I apologized for the way I had spoken to him. We talked a little more, having both calmed down considerably. We went to dinner and had a surprisingly nice time, minus his parking road rage display in the parking lot. Someone beat us to a great parking spot, and he started honking the horn and yelling out the window at two women. I was so mortified. I quickly got out of the car, offering to go get our table at the restaurant. I was praying no one knew I was with him. But the rest of the evening was pleasant. And best of all, I honored my hunger.

> Dear Big Love,
> Adulting can be hard. Relationships can be hard. Please hold me tight.

# 96
## Sadness & Growth

*This morning we talked* more about yesterday's disagreement. I opened up more about my sadness about menopause. I cried a lot in his arms—the kind of crying where I make weird faces and throw lots of tissues on the floor. It felt good. He just listened and patted my hair while I talked about my fear of being old, my sadness about the end of my childbearing years, my depression, my fear that I won't have "it" anymore. It was an intimate time together. I feel grateful for this man in my life. My boobs hurt.

Call to Action: Take a risk and be vulnerable with someone you love today by telling him/her how you really feel.

# 97
# WHAT'S RIGHT WITH ME?

*I went to Toddler Talk.* It was a good review about parenting a toddler and reminded me what a conscientious mother I have been and continue to be. I am so proud of myself at the way I have always sought out parenting resources if/when I realize I don't know what to do. But I also left feeling sad that I don't get to have another baby.

The backs of my knees are sweating. I'm grateful for sweating.

Today marks my anniversary of 20 years of moderate, imperfect eating.

> Dear God,
> Thank You for giving me a good life!

> Call to Action:
> List three things you are doing well right now.

# 98
## Making & Keeping Contracts

*I made an appointment* with a masonry guy to discuss the state of the hardscape in our yard. I rearranged my day and rushed home to accommodate him, and he's still not here three hours later. Where the hell is he? I even washed my hair and put on makeup for him in case he is cute. Something in my armpit keeps itching. Does cancer itch? I'm sure that's what it is. I wish we had some brownies.

10:11 p.m.
I can't sleep. My period ended yesterday, but I still had mild cramps all day today. My foot hurts. I'm preoccupied with whether my son will get into the elementary school I want. When I will find out? TWBD.

> Call to Action:
> Write down a realistic contract you are willing to make and keep today.

Dear God,

For today, I know how much I love myself by the contracts I'm willing to make and keep ... that's what Pat Allen, PhD, reminds her readers. I took time to put things back in their places. Chose reasonably self-loving foods and amounts, and stopped when I was full. I helped a struggling friend on the phone for twenty minutes. I exercised. All these were self-loving acts of faith. The more I do self-loving acts, the more loveable I am. Lovability equals spirituality. Spirituality equals peace of mind.

# Embracing the Little Things

*So today I am still preoccupied* with the yard. Yesterday, the landscape guy (finally) came to discuss the yard. I have never had a yard I chose. I have always just accepted the surroundings that came with the apartment or house I moved into. Now I must sell my husband on the idea. Is there some outfit I can wear that will enhance my landscape presentation to him? I NEED a yard. Could there be feelings I am trying to avoid?

9:25 p.m.
I am still way obsessed with the yard. After putting my son to bed, I flopped on the couch to join my husband sleeping through his second consecutive *Law and Order* rerun on TV. As he snored, I thought I heard the pitter-patter of little feet from afar. I ignored it; wiped out from the day. Thankfully, no mothering requirements resulted, so I forgot about it. I continued watching TV. After watching only half of the episode, I kissed my husband and headed up to bed.

On the way to bed, I checked on my son. I look forward to this every night. His eyes were closed and he was 95 percent asleep. I kissed his cheek and whispered, "I love you," not expecting a response. He mumbled something barely intelligible as he turned to put his other cheek on the pillow.

"What?" I whispered.

He repeated, "Love you too, Mom." Then without ever opening his eyes, he put one hand on his mouth and blew me a kiss. What a gift. This is what I dreamed it'd be like to have a child. I feel so grateful. I am in heaven at this moment. Frosting can't hold a candle to this!

> Dear God,
> Thank You for this boy.

And as if that weren't enough joy for the day, it turned out I hadn't imagined that pitter-patter earlier. Evidently, it had been my son running down to our bedroom just after I'd put him to bed. He placed two of his favorite stuffed animals for my husband and me to sleep with as he often does. Just in case we get scared. My heart is melting. This is the type of thing I live for, and I'm so glad I didn't pad my food today so I could take in every bit of the joy.

> Call to Action:
> List one thing you are grateful for today.

# 100

## Tired[2]

*I woke up warm at 3:00 a.m. today.* I'm restless. Tossed and turned till 4:00 a.m. Woke up again with my husband's alarm at 6:00 a.m. I am so tired. I'm getting the car serviced today, so I dragged myself out of bed.

3:30 p.m.
I am so tired. I have a playdate scheduled with my son and two of his preschool friends and their moms at the park. Ellen DeGeneres' show where she came to our Cardio Dance Party class is supposed to air today. To be completely honest, I'd rather stay home and watch for myself on Ellen and eat frosting, but I'm going to suit up and show up to life and to the park and see what God has planned.

9:00 p.m.
The playdate with the two moms and their sons was fun. They were fun moms to talk to and the kids had a blast running all over the park.

Tonight at dinner, I padded my food a little. I felt sad seeing a friend with her third baby, wishing it were me with the baby instead of my friend. I stopped eating and declared the kitchen closed. I did my nails and I'm going to read in bed now.

> Call to Action: Get horizontal for one minute with the option for longer and then call a supportive friend.

> Dear God,
> Do I really have to go through PM? Isn't this a mistake? I am way too young for this.

# 101

## Sitting Still Through Feelings

*I feel sad about PM today.* I'd really like one more baby. Usually I stay busy to avoid the sadness, but today I just sat still, took a deep breath, and embraced the sadness.

I want to trust that this, too, shall pass. I'd rather eat than trust, but just for one minute I didn't act on that. Not eating is a way to trust God. Trust that I will live through these feelings. I called someone on the PMSS and told them I wanted to eat and what I was feeling.

My friend Cordelia called me back about 20 minutes after I left her a message about my feelings. Thank You, God, and thank you, Cordelia. She pointed out how amazing it is that I have the willingness to identify the feeling of sadness and let myself feel it, rather than eating or staying busy to avoid it. Even though I knew she was right, that didn't make me feel any less sad at first. I got off the phone and sat there a minute, pondering her words. A hint of peace came over me. Not a lot, but I'll take it. The magnitude of what she said started to sink in.

---

**Call to Action:**
Set the timer and sit still for one minute. What comes up?

---

**Reflections:**
How often do I avoid feelings by obsessing on things: what to eat; that pesky chin hair; my to-do list, the stain on the carpet, and my husband's behavior. And how about the yard that must be re-landscaped. And now I'm sweating. Just for today, even if it is just for 10 minutes, I can sit and embrace the feeling of sadness. I rock.

# 102

## Staying Present

*I feel good today.* We had great sex this morning. I felt close to my husband.

I am so glad I didn't eat over my sadness yesterday. It's so worth it today. Even if the feelings come back, which they will.

I led my women's meeting today. I felt quite calm leading the meeting. I was hardly warm at all. I had little negative self-talk. Afterward, I went to lunch with a few friends. Lunch was nice and even though one of the girls at lunch was very annoying, I still enjoyed myself.

A mom friend suggested that I let my son take me on a walk rather than taking him on a walk. This gave me a new insight. Focus on him. What a different perspective. That's why the PMSS is so great. The women in this group encourage each other about the importance of staying present. I'm always thinking whatever I do with him should be elaborate and clever and MOTY-ish. But really, half the time he just wants to be with me while he plays with chopsticks and a plastic lid from a drinking cup. He doesn't require much to entertain him … pinecones, stones, bugs. He's just five, after all.

10:00 p.m.
I was cold today at times! It was exquisite. Leading the meeting was the most relaxed and comfortable and at peace I have ever felt. I wonder if it's because I stayed with the sadness yesterday.

> Dear God,
>
> Please help me to be present with my son and to gracefully balance time with my husband and son. I'm nervous because tomorrow's Sunday, but I know if I stay close to You, I can do anything. TWBD.

# 103

## Sundays – Keep Showing Up

*I was just on the verge* of snapping at my son all day today. His continual fidgeting and challenging of my every word really got on my nerves. I held my tongue. I padded my lunch, but not that much. I think one of the reasons Sundays are so hard, for me, food-wise, is because the pace of the day is different from the others. It's so slow. I am used to full speed ahead with a checklist. I pride myself on being Ms. Efficiency squared. Then Sunday rolls around and there's not much of an agenda. And the whole concept of "family time" still has me somewhat stymied.

I called a PMSS person. After talking with her, I realized I was placing unrealistic expectations on family time. I was thinking family time had to consist of full-blown official activities, such as going to Disneyland. It turns out I've already been doing decent family time without giving myself credit for doing it. So far today we have eaten breakfast at Starbutt's (not the real name), played a board game while there, driven to Target to return something, looked at yard fountains at a garden store and driven to the beach to check the surf and returned home. And all that was before lunch! As is often the case, I was being way too critical of myself. So I backed off Sally and relaxed a little more.

> Dear God,
> Please help me be gentle on myself and to lower my expectations of everything.

# 104
## Critical Voice/ Compassionate Voice: part IV

*I am on an emotional roller coaster today* and it seems like the only way to get off is to overeat. Instead of eating spontaneously, I spent 15 minutes straightening one pile in my home office. I hear Pat Allen's words in my ear: the way out of a negative feeling is a positive decision, followed by action.

*My Critical Voice:*
*Dear Sally,*
*You will never get the yard re-landscaped. Your husband won't go for it. You'll sleep badly tonight because you ate so late tonight. Your son needs to know what school he'll be at. Your book will never even be a book. It's a stupid idea. You are spending too much money lately. You will feel sad about the end of your childbearing years forever.*

*My Compassionate Voice:*
*Dear Sally-Girl,*
*Whether or not the yard gets done is in God's hands. What others think of you or say about you is none of your business. Your stomach was weird tonight. And your food doesn't have to be perfect. And I know you've been waiting for six months to hear about your son's school placement. And that's a long time. Soon you will find out and it'll all work out fine. And your book is fabulous. Just keep writing, against your better judgment.*

*I know you are overwhelmed about it because now you need to put it all in a logical, chronological sequence and add solutions, in between keeping up the house, treating yourself with extreme self-care, being a wife, being a mom, and being an employee. That seems like so much. I know you just want to quit and do nothing but eat. But God will help you with timing and balance. Just keep writing. The journey is the goal.*

*And I know you're disappointed the way your feelings are all over the place today and there's no logical pattern and that's so hard for you. And everything you spent money on is logical, rather than frivolous. It just feels weird because you've stopped feeling guilty for buying stuff like makeup and hair care products; in other words, extreme self-care stuff.*

*Buying a calendar to keep the house running smoothly is not a frivolous purchase. Buying vitamins to keep you and your family healthy is not frivolous. You are trying to run this house and are doing a fantastic job. And yes, you may still feel sad about babies for a long time. And you want to live anyway, I know. One day at a time, with God's help, and sometimes imperfect food.*

*Always remember, God loves you so much He can't take His eyes off you!*

> Call to Action:
> Write your own CV/CV letter and read it to someone you trust.

# 105

## Sleep Becomes a Precious Commodity

*Today my feelings have switched* from high to low so many times I almost didn't write because I couldn't capture my changing feelings on paper fast enough. I forgot about never letting our son sleep with us and had him join us in bed at 2:00 a.m., due to an isolated bed-wetting incident. It seemed like a good idea at the time, since I abhor making his bunk bed. Wrong. Complete sleeplessness ensued for my husband and me because he wiggled and flopped repeatedly, bless his heart.

Operating under sleep-deprived conditions, the day went as follows: I was short with him while getting him ready for school; the extra sheet-washing threw a wrench in my finely tuned routine. I didn't feel so great about my parenting skills. The good news is, I apologized. After dropping him off, I called a PMSS member crying because I can't take this waiting to know if he got switched to the elementary school I want for another second.

Then the gym was great. Another guy said good morning and class was dreamy with my handsome Cardio Dance Party instructor, as usual.

I dropped off the old Cox modem at a UPS Store and bought two birthday cards. Efficiency excites me!

I cried about the kindergarten saga to another PMSS member. I had a relaxing facial.

I didn't get to work on the book as much as I had hoped. I have cramps.

> Dear God,
> Please give me the ability to take each day as it comes. I want the ability to wear each day like a loose garment. To love myself and those around me, no matter how the day unfolds. To give the reins back to You. But please could You help me get some sleep tonight?

# 106

## Public Speaking

*Today was a great day.* I unexpectedly spoke at my women's meeting because someone was out. I'm just proud of myself for letting God speak through me. After the meeting, I went to the Sawdust Festival with my son, Cordelia (45), and her two kids. It was hard to decide whether to go or not, but it ended up being fun. I really enjoyed it. My son got a toe ring. My food was self-loving. The kids all had fun.

I really enjoyed watching jive dancing and mambo dancing on TV tonight. There's something very sensual about them both. I love that. Maybe I'm ovulating. Note to self: Explore jive and/or mambo dance lessons.

I loved being in my body today. I felt sexy. I felt sensually aware. I loved it. I felt alive and present. I got more Victoria's Secret bras in four colors and panties to match. Maybe it's the inner Victoria's Secret in me talking.

10:30 p.m.
I am so happy I can't even sleep. I tend to have one day in my cycle like this where I am completely euphoric and today was that day. Food didn't call my name. I got a note from a dear friend today, saying she loves our talks and I inspire her. It added to my day's happiness. I feel so cute and empowered and complete. I feel really horny. How exciting. I thought I'd never feel like that again. It's sort of like a "Green Light" day, only better. I loved making eye contact with people all day today. I almost didn't write about this because I feel so sure that these feelings will be with me forever. But I did anyway because this, too, shall pass!

> *Dear Sally-Girl,*
> *Wasn't it wonderful to be so calm and feel so relaxed and content with your public-speaking challenge ... and be cute, too? And isn't it wonderful to be able to turn this over (fear of public speaking) to God at a new level lately. I know you are excited about that because it's something you've never been able to do. You've always known you had so many wonderful thoughts to convey, but couldn't access them while speaking. And somehow, you've tapped into the Source in these past two weeks. You deserve to be happy about your accomplishment. And you're such a great parent, too.*
> *Love, Big Love*

# 107
## One Load of Laundry a Day Keeps the Basketball Away

*My friend Cordelia* has urged me to subscribe to the free website service called Flylady.net. This woman, "Fly Lady," has dedicated her life to helping women declutter their homes. Although her decluttering campaign covers a host of domestic areas, from shining your kitchen sink to dressing all the way to your shoes, my favorite idea is her laundry suggestion. Every night before bed, I put one load of laundry in the washer, without starting it. The following morning upon awakening, I put in the soap and turn on the washer. By the time I have gotten dressed (sometimes) all the way to the shoes, made the bed and come downstairs, the load is ready for the dryer. Then, little by little throughout the day, I fold that ONE load and put it away.

Reflections:
Dr. Pat Allen's words guide me: I know how much I love myself by the contracts I am willing to make and keep. The more I love myself, the more often I choose nutritional foods and amounts.

Call to Action: Decide on one contract item you are willing to make and keep today.

# 108

## Writing is Healing

*Here I am, awake with cramps.* Aside from that, I'm lying here contemplating how much progress I have made in the areas of self-acceptance and self-love. I've used several powerful writing tools for years to help counteract my proclivity to negative self-talk. Although these exercises always bring me great relief, my negative self-talk still creeps back at times. But lately, I've had a lot more clarity on this.

It's hard to explain. It's a shift I can detect in my perspective about life … an improvement. I have this peace about me … a sort of blanket self-acceptance that I don't usually have. It's more than acceptance. It's like self-excitement and love! Could this be what the menopause authors mean when they talk about something good coming out of menopause? I still haven't opened my menopause book, but I read the back cover.

Could this seeming spiritual shift in perspective be a result of menopause? Part of me doesn't even want to acknowledge that, because that means I'm accepting PM and another part of me still wants to kick and scream about PM. Yet I can't deny how content I feel at this moment. We'll see. Guess I could write about it. For now, I'll put a pillow under my knees and continue to ponder. And to think I've already finished washing my one daily load of laundry. TWBD.

> Dear God,
> Thank You for the ability to be open-minded and aware as I grow and change for the better.

# 109

## Spontaneous Eating/Staying Current with Feelings

12:30 p.m.
I just spontaneously ate a cookie with my lunch because I must go to my staff meeting for work. That means I will have to go back to work soon. Ewww. I don't ever want to go back. I love being off the clock. Funny how eating the cookie didn't make the situation go away. Now I still feel sad about the imminence of returning to work AND I have a slight sugar high. Not worth it. At least I feel cute and two men said hi to me at the gym earlier. I will suit up and show up to the staff meeting and my lunch is over. The kitchen is closed, against my better judgment. LOL.

I am willing to write a very brief letter to Big Love and have Big Love write back a short reply. This writing exercise helps me stay current with my feelings, so I eat spontaneously less often.

*Dear Big Love,*
*I feel resentful because I have committed to return to work when I would rather stay home. But I know how much I love myself by the contracts I'm willing to make and keep. Dammit.*
*Love, Sally*

Call to Action:
Write a one-sentence Letter to God (Universe, Big Love, Nature) and have Him/Her write you back with a one-sentence letter, with the option to write more. This will help you stay current with your feelings.

Dear [insert name of your higher power here],
I feel [BLANK] because [BLANK]...
Love, [your name here]

Dear [your name here],
"higher power" replies to your letter using one sentence.
Love, [higher power name here]

*Dear Sally-Girl,*
*I know you don't want to go. I know you are super tired. I know you are a morning person and not a late-afternoon person. I love you anyway. Do you think this commitment was too big a commitment for you? Next time, let's review before we make this one again.*
*Love, Big Love*

# 110

## Writing and Reading Aloud:
### your cv/cv letters are powerful

*Here I am, awake with cramps again.* I had a load in the washer already from last night, so I went downstairs and started the washer. I got back in bed. I still feel great emotionally and spiritually, I guess, mostly because I'm having this moment of clarity, as my old friend Cordelia used to say. For years, I've known that I give too much power to what other people think of me. When I do that, the price is decreased serenity. Yet even though I've worked to overcome this tendency, and made lots of progress, I've never been able to stop completely.

Whenever I do it, I stop and write myself two letters. In the first letter, I really let my head go wild. I put all the mean things my head's saying to me on paper … really. Just to get it all out. Such as, "No one likes you at work. They all think you're stupid" (critical voice/CV). Next, I write another letter to myself, and I let myself off the hook (compassionate voice/CV). In this letter I dissect the first letter, line by line, and counter every sentence with a self-loving statement.

Now, I love rules. The rules of this writing exercise are that the second letter must always be written at the same sitting as the first letter and be of equal length or longer than the first letter. Whereas the first letter is from my dark side, to me, the second letter is from my Higher Self or God, to me. Then I call one of my PMSS buddies and read both letters aloud to her on the phone. It's very healing … very powerful.

> **Call to Action:**
> Check in with yourself. Is there any negative self-talk (NST) going on inside your head right now? If you're not sure, notice if non-nutritious food choices are calling your name from the kitchen. If they are, then chances are you have some NST going on. Try the CV/CV writing exercise at this junction on an NST issue you are dealing with. You've got nothing to lose except some of those voices that are holding you back.

# III

## Intimacy

*My husband's taking the day off.* That's really going to cramp my style. My son will be in preschool. I was looking forward to being alone all day. Against my better judgment, I have opted to go to the beach with him in lieu of my original plan, which consisted of Group Cardio at the gym, grocery shopping, and paying bills. I know it sounds crazy, but I love my routine. TWBD.

> Dear God,
> Help me let go of my rigidity.

# 112

## Blow Jobs and Board Meetings

*Getting connected to my husband* amidst his rigorous work schedule can be a challenge. He is frequently exhausted and, quite understandably, all he wants to do is zone out or sleep. We ended up having a really nice time together today. I came up with an idea he could relate to. I told him we were having a Board Meeting. I said, "Honey, now I am giving my report as the Director of Parenting" and got him up to speed on our son's latest behavioral adventures. Next, I switched to Director of Bill-Paying, then Director of Landscape Architecture, then to Director of Spiritual Growth.

It obviously worked because he engaged in conversation with me. At the end of our chat, I indicated how good I feel when we can talk to each other, without interruptions. I asked him what the secret is to get him to talk like that. He said, "A blow job." If my husband is nothing else, he is direct.

> Dear God,
> Thank You for Your help.

# 113
## Too Much Intimacy

*I made the mistake* of reading an excerpt from my journal to my husband yesterday. After that, I never wanted to write again. But I am writing anyway. I am already dreading tomorrow because Sunday is family day and they're so hard for me. I feel lonely. I can't figure out how to "do" family time. I need to figure out what I want to do.

> *10:00 p.m.*
> *My Critical Voice:*
> *Sally,*
> *You were so stupid to eat spontaneously tonight … and stupid to read your journal to your husband. And stupid to think you could write a book. Your husband doesn't think you can do it. And you know you can't. And your son won't get into the elementary school you want him to go to. And it's so stupid that you don't know how to do the weekend with your family, when having a family was*

*all you ever wanted in life. You are old and have a big middle.*

My Compassionate V*oice:*
*Dear Sally-Girl,*
*I love you. no matter what you eat. You are a compulsive eater and sometimes you overeat. I always love you. Don't let your husband's opinion change yours. Sometimes I think he's afraid to be supportive of you because he's jealous; afraid you'll replace him. Perhaps it was a mistake to share with him, but your heart was in the right place. You were trying to be close. The writing you shared with him was probably one of the most poignant collection of words you've put to paper. It might have plain gone over his head. It's not important what your husband thinks about the book. He's not menopausal and never will be. And the book's successful publishing does not hinge on his support or his approval. This is about you getting on with your life and accepting what is ... and embracing menopause.*

*And your son will get into just the right school for him. And how would you know how to do family time? You were the youngest in your family and there wasn't much family life because your siblings were so much older than you. You'll learn how to handle family time! You're overdue for a New Wave Day and your weight is fine. I know there are a lot of things you're waiting for right now: When will your husband's surgery be? When will you hear which school your son will be going to for kindergarten?*

*And I know the sadness over no second baby is intensified with each twinge of cramps and boobs hurting … and with each pregnant woman sighting. I know that sadness seems endless.*

Always remember, God loves you so much He can't take His eyes off you!

# 114
## Too Sad

*I feel tired and depressed.* I don't want to write because I don't want to be going through menopause. It's too sad. Maybe I should just call the whole thing off. Hopefully, tomorrow I won't be sad.

> Reflection:
> I enjoy writing. It is an escape for me. I believe that tomorrow will be a better day. I want to live, no matter what.

# 115

## Self-Esteem Takes a Beating ... and (Hopefully) Keeps on Ticking

*Every so often, I feel down.* I doubt everything about myself. Today is yet another one of those days. I do not want to be PM. I found a gray hair while blow-drying today. I feel old. I feel huge. I feel unattractive. I don't want to write. I want to quit. I just want to eat frosted things.

9:30 p.m.
I am so glad I chose self-loving foods over frosting today. I've had minor cramps on and off all day.

> Dear God,
> Help me remember to trust You and to have enough patience to wait for answers without eating. And help me to remember that eating isn't a remedy for my bouts of sadness or my perimenopause.

# 116
## Dessert Day

*As I have mentioned,* I have been maintaining a 35-lb. weight loss for over 30 years. I eat a lot of vegetables daily. I exercise 3-5 times per week. I am willing to limit my portion sizes most of the time rather than eat with wild abandon because I feel better when I do that. One of the ways I keep my weight off is by making sure I never feel deprived. So even though my intake of sugary, high-fat food is minimal daily, I must give myself a break occasionally. One of the breaks I give myself is a weekly Dessert Day.

Once a week, I purchase the most delicious dessert I can think of. I have done this for years. The onset of acid reflux necessitated I limit chocolate consumption. Therefore, Dessert Day became Brownie Day for a while (yes, I know that brownies are chocolate, but I don't expect perfection from myself), but, all in all, Dessert Day continues to work fine for me. I love identifying behaviors and naming them. I also love rituals, so I make one out of this, too. I always have an ice-cold glass of milk with it and eat it as slowly as possible, enjoying every bite.

> Reflections:
> One dessert a week does not a Basketball make. I'm grateful for the gift of eating in moderation.

# 117
## Dessert Day Malfunction

*I am a little embarrassed to admit* that I made two trips to Paradise Bakery today to get THE BROWNIE. Both times, I was told they weren't finished frosting them yet and to come back in an hour. So, reluctantly, I bought a piece of carrot cake instead. My vanity wouldn't permit me to make a third trip to the bakery in the same day. Mind you, their carrot cake is outstanding, especially regarding the ample frosting-to-cake ratio. But you know when you just have "chocolate anticipation" indelibly imprinted on your taste buds around the 21st day of your menstrual cycle? Well then you know that even carrot cake with frosting two inches thick—which theirs isn't!—just won't cut it. So about five hours after eating the carrot cake, I reached for two sugar cookies with pink frosting that we just happened to have left over from Sunday's New Wave Day. Then those were followed by some honey-roasted peanuts, just so the protein food group wouldn't feel left out.

Tonight I feel huge. I made non-nutritional food choices spontaneously. What are the feelings I'm attempting to avoid by excess food? I am not in touch with them right now, but I know that they will surface within the next 24-48 hours if I stay present to the best of my ability. Meanwhile, I'm at that point in my menstrual cycle where I feel big, no matter what I eat anyway. My clothes feel tighter. Even my fabulous Victoria's Secret bras feel tighter. So, I figured I might as well eat pink frosted cookies. Some days that's the best I can do.

*Dear Paradise Bakery: get your f-ing act together with the brownies, you idiots!*

*Dear Son: stop wiggling. And stop making gibberish sounds. You are driving me crazy!*

I know from how annoyed I am with everything that the bad time of the month is definitely here. Oh … crap.

> Dear God,
> Please slow me down so I can get in touch with what I am feeling and give me the willingness to sit with it. Please give me the ability to get comfortable with feeling uncomfortable.

# 118

## I Am Huge! I Got the Basketball Overnight!

*I am in the PMS time of my cycle right now.* I feel huge and I am not really eating more than I usually eat. But having this bloated feeling makes me feel big, and then I reason that I just might as well overeat because I feel big anyway. I might as well at least enjoy some non-nutritional food while I'm at it. I have taken extra time to prepare large portions of veggie-laden dishes today to help me get through this time. This is the part of PM I hate. It'll be at least a week before I get my period, and I am already experiencing symptoms. I was awakened at 3:00 a.m. today with cramps. This has been happening each cycle for the past five cycles now. And my boobs hurt.

I obsessed on THE BROWNIES on and off all day today. Finally, I called the bakery and asked them to put one aside for me and I drove over and picked it up. I didn't eat it. Just having it in the bag made me feel better. Maybe later. After I picked my son up from preschool, we went to Cordelia's house so our kids could play and I could flat-iron Cordelia's hair (I am on a mission to flat-iron all my curly, frizzy-haired sisters so they can experience the same high I do after suffering with the hair trauma for life).

After Cordelia's hair liberation, she and her kids walked my son and me home in the still-warm summer air. It was what I call a perfect family moment. The sun was just going down as we met up with my husband washing his car in the driveway. Several other neighbors were out walking, and we were all greeting each other. This is the life I always dreamed of. I was so happy at that moment I didn't even care that my boobs hurt.

> Dear God,
> Help me remember what is important. Help me remember to take my eyes off what I look like for just one moment today and notice the blessings around me.

# 119
## Feelings Will NOT Kill Me

*I just dropped my son off* for his last day of preschool. I am feeling a surge of various conflicting emotions simultaneously. Sad that he won't be at this preschool anymore that has taken such loving care of my only child for an entire year. Excited to see where his next chapter in life will take him. And here come the tears as I write this. Now I realize what the past two-day brownie obsession has been about. I was trying not to feel this. I guess I am ready to feel it now. I also feel proud of myself and my husband for the good job we are doing raising him, even though it's imperfect. I feel amazed at how far my son has come emotionally, mentally, developmentally, and spiritually. And I'm proud of how far I have come: emotionally, mentally, and spiritually as a mother, a wife, and a sassy woman!

Looking back at these last five years, I have walked through fears time and time again, without excess food and sometimes with excess food. But 75 percent of the time I don't eat excess food because of my faith and willingness to commit to extreme self-care. I have made boundaries that I thought would literally kill me if I stuck to them—yet lived to tell about it. I've said "No" to my son hundreds of times and stuck to it. Being a mom is the thing I wanted most in life. Little did I know it would also be the hardest thing I'd ever done. Yet here I am doing it at 45 years old, and feeling surprisingly good about myself. It felt good to cry these tears of joy. I just knew there were feelings behind that affair I was having with the brownie. Sometimes I am so adorable I just can't stand it, especially when my hair is flat-ironed … but even when it's not.

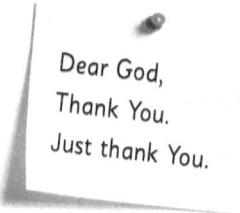

Dear God,
Thank You.
Just thank You.

# 120

## Lotion Works Miracles

*My son spent the night at his aunt's house.* It wasn't long enough! I just want to eat. I was judgmental of everyone I encountered today. I got Basketball stomach overnight and I haven't even eaten spontaneously in a few days. Well, not since the whole Dessert-Day-malfunction ordeal, anyway. I feel bloated and huge. I hate everyone. Nothing and no one is enough. My husband is at the beach all day. It's too hot. I just want to sleep all day. I don't want to be responsible for another person at all today.

8:48 p.m.
I just finished the witching hour. Today is only day 24 of my cycle and it's an "Everyone-Just-F-ing-Get-Away-From-Me" day. My fingernails are even getting on my nerves. So are the in-betweens of my teeth. I took a shower with some aromatherapy scrubby thing. I smell great. After that, I put

on lotion and I got eye cream in my eye and it stings like crazy. I must write this with one eye closed and watering. It all seems like the end of the world. And now my zit count is up to five. Now I must make it through another six days (assuming this cycle will be my "old" typical length) of this.

> Dear God,
> I am really going to need Your help, please. I am sure I have a full-blown Basketball right now.
> TWBD.

# 121

## Special Encore Performance: basketball paranoia, sundays are the worst, murder/death/kill, everyone-just-get-away-from-me! medley

*We had a family beach day today.* I packed self-loving food choices for all of us before leaving. It takes a little longer, but I am worth it.

I surfed. I've come to realize that surfing isn't about catching waves for me right now, though it may be later in my life. Right now, it's about me getting into the water to get a break from being mom and wife, a break from worries, Basketball paranoia, whatever. I am at the mercy of the surf, and it's therefore impossible to obsess on Basketball or anything else for that matter. It's just God and me out there and

I talk out loud to Him and paddle my brains out, fighting just to stay on the board. It was a real perspective-gainer. My fatigued body feels tired but wonderful. And to think, there's only one hour left of the witching hour. Woo Hoo! And Cordelia's bringing her kids over to play with my son while I flat-iron her hair again.

> Dear God,
> Thank You for perspective.
> Thank You for the ocean.
> Thank You for flat irons.

# 122

## Dear God, I Feel…

*Dear God,*
*I feel overwhelmed. Here we go. My son didn't get into the elementary school I wanted him to go to. I took him to meet his kindergarten teacher today. Will my son have a good experience at this school … with this teacher? The not-knowing makes me anxious. I know it'll all work out. But can't I just know NOW!? I just want to eat right now. Just for the next five minutes, I won't act on that impulse. It's so hard not knowing. I have cramps and my boobs hurt and that's not helping anything. I'm worried about work starting, even though that's still seven days away. I'm tired. I don't want my son ever to grow up.*

4:00 p.m.
I called Cordelia complaining about my husband. My husband is a full-day beach-loving person. I am a partial-day beach person. I was still ruminating about Sunday's beach

jaunt, 24 hours after the fact. As I was venting my discontent about my husband in one area, it led to another beef about him. My husband has not been helping to keep the home organized. Getting our home organized was one of the primary concerns he voiced in marriage counseling approximately one year ago. Cordelia suggested I call our marriage & family therapist for what I call a marriage "tune-up." In talking things out with these two women, I realized my part in all this: I have not stayed current in my communication with my husband. I often forget he can't read my mind. With the guidance of a safe friend and a trained professional, I planned out in written form what I wanted to say to him to address these situations in a healthy, normal, and appropriate way. I haven't even read him my stuff yet, but already I feel much better. I feel ready to face the witching hour!

Sunday Beach Boundary: Two hours max or take two cars.

Dear Universe,
Please give me the ability to let go of what my body looks like and love myself on the inside. And remind me that You love me so much.

9:31 p.m.
The witching hour went okay. I didn't answer when the food called me. Even though my food choices were nutritional and my portions self-loving, I still feel like I'm sporting the Basketball. I'm just going to put that in the hands of the Universe for right now and go to sleep.

# 123

## Sleep

*I couldn't sleep last night.* I was restless. Oh … no wonder … my period began at 4:00 this afternoon. I feel so sad about my period having come as I always do. I feel like my body is gigantic. I feel BBB (beyond Basketball big). Yet my food choices were nutritional and my portions sizes self-loving. When I still feel huge after having made self-loving food choices, I really want to throw in the towel and mow through some food. I thought about serious quantity-eating today and decided not to act on the thoughts. I'll trust that these sad (and basketball) feelings will pass. I'm going to bed now.

> Dear God,
> Please give me sleep—soon and sound. TWBD.

# 124
## Fall/Winter Clothing Denise-ification Day

*Today my period was the heaviest flow* I have ever had. They are the worst prolonged cramps I've ever had except that one period five months ago when this whole PM came to my attention in the first place. And I am even doing the Motrin trick. I just wanted to sit down all day. And I would have, except for the fact that I was clothes-shopping for the fall and winter season.

I kept my food choices nutritional and my portions self-loving, even though I feel huge and Basketball-prone. What's the point?

My husband has been approached by a headhunter about a job in Hawaii. For him, it'd be a dream come true to live in the Aloha State. Not so much, though, for this freckled redhead who, as of late, avoids all heat like the plague. And we're not even addressing leaving my dear

MOTY Club; my PMSS friends; the job I love; the school district I love; and the relatively low humidity my otherwise frizzy hair loves.

Of course, these types of prospective job offers take weeks till they get even remotely close to coming to fruition, but a small area of my brain is busily projecting about what it would all look like living in Hawaii as I write and endure my beloved cramps. In fact, I am so adept at projecting that I am near tears, just picturing my son and me eating dinner alone, crying because I miss my life and straight hair in Southern California so much. And of course, I am sweating, and I have the Basketball in this vivid Hawaiian mental image. And I have skin cancer.

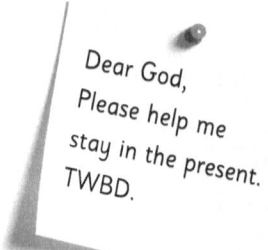

Dear God,
Please help me stay in the present.
TWBD.

# 125

## Spend More Time Being "Unproductive"

*I struck up a conversation* with a young woman in the locker room at the gym this morning. I was attracted to her because she was flat-ironing her hair and I wanted to glean from "her any flat-ironing pearls of wisdom she might possess. It turned out our flat-iron knowledge was about equal; however, we formed an immediate flat-iron bond when she offered, "You know, I came into the gym to work out today, but found I was just too tired. I decided the best thing to do was to iron my hair instead." I gave her a knowing smile as I enthusiastically responded, "Yes, I get it!"

I am grateful to this young woman whose name I don't even know because she did teach me something, albeit not about ironing technique. I adore ironing my hair, but often I feel like I shouldn't spend 30+ minutes blow-drying/ironing it because it's frivolous. She taught me that spending extra time to style my hair in a way that makes me feel pretty is time well spent. In effect, she gave me permission to be what I would define as unproductive to feel better. Thank you!

> Dear God,
> Please help me reassess the value of being unproductive. Please give me the ability to reframe self-care as something desirable instead of something to criticize.

> Call to Action:
> Think of a self-care behavior that you avoid because your head says it is a waste of time. Rethink your self-talk around it.

# 126

## Dessert Day Malfunction Follow-Up

*Yesterday I called Paradise Bakery* before driving over for "THE Brownie" since they didn't have any brownies last Wednesday. I got the manager, Tracey, on the phone. She apologized, saying there was a problem with the chocolate supplier and there would be no brownies again that day. I was somewhat shocked by what happened next. "But I know exactly who you are," she said. She continued "You're the one who comes for a brownie every Wednesday. We are so sorry about last week and now again today. Please come back tomorrow and we will give you two free brownies. We know how important a chocolate fix can be."

> Dear God,
> Thank You for Tracey … today's PM angel!

OMG! Sometimes I just LOVE people! I went back today, and she rose to the occasion. I was so impressed I emailed a letter of praise to Tracey's employer. Maybe Tracey understands PM.

> Call to Action:
> Write a note or letter to someone to tell that person what's RIGHT with him or her.

# 127
## Yearly Cumulative "Great Things Dad's Done" List

*Unfortunately, blemishing my husband* comes much more naturally to me than praising him. The good news is, I am committed to positive progress in this area. I learned a helpful tool from a mom in my local chapter of the MOMS (Moms Offering Moms Support) Club. It's called the "Great Things Dad's Done" list. I keep a journal for our son about his life. I write down funny things our son says and every few months I write down what his typical day consists of—random musings about him.

I also keep a page marked to record precious things my husband does for our son. Like the morning he stopped and put our son's train track back together at 6:00 a.m. while getting ready to drive two hours for an important meeting at work. Then there was the day my husband took the entire day off work to be present at our son's parent-teacher conference for preschool. On Father's Day, I rewrite the list inside of his Father's Day card as one way of showing my appreciation for what a great dad he is.

> Reflection:
> Do we need to start the alpha chapter of MMOMMS Club (Menopausal Moms Offering Menopausal Moms Support)?

> Call to Action:
> Start a chapter in your area.

# 128
## "Economizing" on Feelings

*Even though I know* it is vital to my well-being to do so, I will do just about anything not to feel my feelings. One of my many tactics is what I like to call "economizing on feelings." Economizing on feelings is when I try to force myself to feel multiple feelings all at the same time before they are present. Another similar tactic is "pre-feeling." This is when I predict a certain feeling will be coming soon (example: I will be sad when my mom dies). I try to pre-feel it, to get it out of the way sooner.

The bottom line: it's impossible to economize on or pre-feel feelings. They cannot be scheduled. They cannot be planned for 9:00 p.m. tomorrow night when I have already removed my makeup. They will come up when they want to and if I don't let them come up, I tend to have a bigger appetite. And we all know, bigger appetites can lead to bigger portions and bigger portions lead to Basketballs. Or so my Critical Voice says.

> Dear God,
> Please give me the willingness and the ability to live life on life's terms ... to relax and let go of the timing of my feelings.

# 129
## From Sadness to a Blessing

*I have worked* in the fitness industry for many years. My career choice was heavily influenced by the experiences of my mother. From the time I was a young girl, my mother lived with chronic pain. As soon as one health condition went away, another replaced that one. Her pain reduced her activity level and significantly diminished the quality of her life. Her pain also reduced her availability to participate in my life. Sadly, although she tried endless solutions, she was practically never pain-free for most of my life. As a result, at a young age I vowed never to allow my life to become so small and inactive. I resolved to stay as physically, intellectually, emotionally, and spiritually fit as possible and to pass that on to others in any way I could. I am thankful for this situation because it remains today my greatest passion to help others live their best life. Thank you, Mom. I love you.

> Dear God,
> Please give me courage to let myself walk through the uncomfortable and/or sad feelings today.

# 130

## Walking Through Fears Is My PM Antidrug

*Years ago,* my career in fitness began as a personal trainer. I was credentialed many times over. I knew the body, and I have always been solid with one-on-one communication. As things evolved, I began to receive offers to teach group exercise classes. I turned them down because I had a huge fear of public speaking—HUGE. As in extreme stomach upset, sleeplessness, and anxiety off the charts. My perfectionism and my need to engage in "impression management" played a large role in keeping my life small. As opportunities continued to present themselves, I realized I needed to walk through my fears. How could I keep my commitment to be physically, intellectually, emotionally, and spiritually fit and inspire the world to do the same if I hid behind my fear? I had to walk the talk. I affirmed my willingness to accept the next offer I received. Not long after, the next offer came to me. It was from a community college to teach a class of about 100 adults over 50 years of age … on a stage … with a microphone. I heard someone say, "Yes, I'd love the opportunity. Thank you for asking [Gulp]." That someone was me.

Even though I was extremely nervous, I set out to learn how to teach group fitness. With little public speaking experience and no dance background whatsoever, I began to watch videos, take notes, and practice. I studied for and passed a group fitness certification exam. I took dance lessons. Basically, I memorized enough material to teach one class session.

The first day of class approached. My biggest fear was completely blanking in front of 100 strangers. My second biggest fear was that I'd be criticized for not having enough dance moves. Both fears came true on the first day of class. But I got through it. Over time, I received more compliments than criticisms.

Music combined with physical movement can be healing on physical, intellectual, and emotional levels, especially for adults over 50 (which I am now, too). If I had not stepped out of my comfort zone and walked through my fear, I would never have discovered that.

Further, the high I experienced because of having walked through a huge personal fear was indescribable.

Walking through fears ... who knew?

> Dear God,
> Please give me courage to let myself walk through the uncomfortable today.

Call to Action:
List the action that keeps calling your name that you are too fearful to attempt. Be willing to walk through this to get to the other splendid, free, empowered side.

# 131
## Discover What Makes Your Heart Sing and DO It!

*"I know how much I love myself by the contracts
I'm willing to make and keep."*
–Patricia Allen, PhD

*Challenge yourself* physically, intellectually, emotionally, and spiritually

*Past Endeavors:*
2004: Published article in *IDEA Health & Fitness Source Magazine* on walking through insecurities professionally to build self-confidence

2006 – Present: STOTT Pilates Certification (huge physical and intellectual challenge)

2011 – Present: Learned and daily use QuickBooks (intellectual and spiritual)

2012 – Present: beading/macramé work (spiritual)

2012-2015 – Earned black belt in taekwon-do with my son (physical, intellectual, spiritual)

2013 – Helped plan and throw Cordelia's daughter's Country Bling Sweet 16 Party

2015 – Published article in CSUF's Center for Successful Aging newsletter on how adults over 50 benefit from practicing Pilates

2015 – Presented workshop at CSUF's Annual Successful Aging Conference

2015 – Present: MELT Method certification and daily use (physical, intellectual, emotional, spiritual)

2017 – Completed 4-unit and 3-unit, transferrable Accounting and QuickBooks courses, respectively, at community college at age 57.

1984 – Present: Journal writing about feelings; about relationships; affirmations; about healing and staying current; and about menopause.

2005 – Present: Wrote and published a book that empowers women to unite and navigate perimenopause and beyond, Physically + Intellectually + Emotionally + Spiritually

2020: Published in *IDEA Fitness Journal* Member Spotlight on giving back to the community on social media during turbulent times

*Current Endeavors:*
2019 – Present: Online and in-person courses and retreats that empower and unite women to achieve clarity and confidence about their second chapter of life: Physically + Intellectually + Emotionally + Spiritually

> Dear Universe,
> Help me be open to exploring things that feel scary to me that I may truly discover the purpose You have in mind for me.

> Romans 12:2 (The Living Bible)
> Don't copy the behavior and customs of this world but be a new and different person with a fresh newness in all you do and think. Then you will learn from your own experience how His ways will really satisfy you.

# 132

## LISTEN TO WHAT MAKES YOUR HEART SING

*As a fitness professional,* I attend huge fitness conferences yearly that offer every type of fitness class under the sun. I have always enjoyed trying all types of exercise classes offered at these conferences … except one. There was one type of exercise I had never tried because I was sure I wouldn't like it. Pilates. I had all sorts of preconceived ideas about what it was and what it wasn't, so I was sure it was not for me. Basically, I had contempt prior to investigation.

One day, my handsome Cardio Dance Party instructor told our class he had attended a Pilates instructor-training workshop and loved it. Well, not only did I find him easy on the eyes, I also highly respected his opinions about fitness. Basically, if he endorsed it, count me in. I immediately began researching Pilates instructor-training programs and soon my training was underway. After years of strength training, practicing Pilates was like nothing I had ever experienced. It was simultaneously invigorating, not only physically but also mentally challenging, and relieved stress. Further, I felt better and my clothes fit differently … in a good way. My Pilates journey began that continues to this day. In short, Pilates makes my heart sing.

> Dear God,
> Please open my mind to try new things. Help me keep my eyes open for something that may unexpectedly make my heart sing.

# 133

## TRY SOMETHING NEW, EVEN IF YOU KNOW YOU'RE GONNA HATE IT

*Originally,* I had planned to attend only one Pilates course, to prove to myself that I was right and that I would hate it. Surprise. Once I tried it, I fell in love with it, and my plan changed. I soon realized that learning how to practice it correctly and teach Pilates was quite an undertaking. The certifying organization I chose had very rigorous standards for certification. Preparation for each level and type of certification required hundreds of hours of coursework, studying, observation, and practice teaching, not to mention both written and oral exams covering anatomy, human movement, and postural analysis. That meant a lot of focus and memorization. Based on my PM experiences about my ability to focus and memorize up to this time, I seriously

> Dear God,
> Please give me the willingness to try something I think I'll hate. Give me the courage to open my mind. I may hate it ... but I may not hate it. And it may impact my life for the better on the cellular level.

questioned whether I was up to the task. Yet my piqued interest urged me forward.

I didn't let my fears stop me. I developed an elaborate system of color-coded flash cards from which to study and carried them with me everywhere. It was a multiple-year process. As soon as my son learned to read, I even had him use the flash cards to quiz me when we were on long drives. One step at a time, I diligently, patiently made my way through each course and its requirements. Over the next four years, I successfully completed every type of Pilates instructor certification that my chosen certifying organization offered, from essential to advanced levels.

Just as I expected, earning my Pilates certifications greatly increased my career skill set and gave me a new activity that made my heart sing. What I hadn't expected was that in the process of learning Pilates, my previously waning self-confidence would be restored to full capacity. I realized to my great relief, I still had a brain and I still know how to use it! Thank you, Pilates.

I am so glad I opened my mind to Pilates, against my "better" judgment.

Call to Action:

Is there something you just "know" you will hate that keeps calling your name? List it on paper and send it up to God or out to the Universe.

# 134
## Outdoor Cycling Makes My Heart Sing

*I have always loved to ride my bicycle.* I prefer to ride outdoors. I don't ride a street bike; I ride a mountain bike in the street. I like the fat tires. I like to be upright. It just works for me. In 1999, I fulfilled a personal goal of participating in a 100-mile bike ride (the Solvang Century) on my mountain bike. By the time I pedaled across the finish line, all the celebration booths were pretty much cleaned up and no one was around to cheer for me, but I finished! Who cares? I was ecstatic. I trained. I finished.

Not long after that I joyfully learned I was pregnant with my first and only child, just as I turned 40. I rarely bicycled again for the next several years. Sure, I still worked out, in between motherhood joys, but like most mothers, I struggled to fit everything in. Besides, I had aspired to ride one, not multiple centuries. Then one day, for some random reason, I rode my bike again. It dawned on me … I LOVE riding my bike outdoors. It makes my heart sing. What am I waiting for? From that moment of clarity on, I have pretty much ridden my bicycle outside every Monday for about 30 minutes. It's not a super-long ride, and sometimes I ride more than just on Monday. But just knowing that once a week, I get to feel the breeze in my face, hear the birds sing and feel that pure joy boosts my immune system immeasurably.

Reflection:
Is there anything that makes my heart sing that I have been putting off because I just don't have time for Olympic-caliber participation … or for no apparent reason? I want to be willing to make time for whatever it is and do it now. Just for today.

Call to Action:
Has a small voice been calling you lately to participate in an activity you love? Listen to that voice … it knows.

# 135
## Beading Makes My Heart Sing

*From the time I was 8 or 9 years of age,* I loved crafts. I was particularly into making macramé plant holders and bracelets. I even made macramé wall hangings, belts, and purses. As a preteen, I was selling my work at a craft fair. I once sold so much macramé that I made enough money to buy myself my first Schwinn 10-speed bicycle, a bright orange Schwinn Varsity. Then as a teen, my interests shifted from crafts and macramé to other things.

Until about eight years ago, I hadn't given my craftiness a thought. Then one day, I received an email advertisement for something called a "wrap bracelet." I admired it. I love to wear bracelets, but sometimes have a hard time finding them in colors I like. Out of the blue, remembering my crafty days, I said to myself, "I could make that, and I could make it in colors I love." I googled around and found a website that sold beading materials and provided tutorials.

Now I have a cupboard for my beading supplies, thanks to the Denise-ification. I have made more than 100 bracelets and putting together each one made my heart sing. Beading is therapeutic and relaxing for me.

> Call to Action:
> Think about some project or activity that you loved doing as a child that you might want to revisit.

# 136
## Contempt Prior to Investigation and the MELT Method

*As I've mentioned,* I yearly attend a huge fitness conference to earn continuing education credits. It is an opportunity to learn firsthand about the latest research in fitness. In 2013, my fitness-BFF Cordelia (then 43) urged me to attend a workshop about something called the MELT Method. She said it would be about fascia. I didn't really understand what the word *fascia* meant, but I really like to be with Cordelia and I only see her once a year at these conferences, so I agreed to join her.

The MELT Method is a simple self-treatment technique to restore health and balance in the myofascial (myo = muscle, fascia = connective tissue), nervous, and lymphatic systems of the body using a soft foam roller and rubber balls of varying sizes and densities. In the workshop, we learned that MELT techniques balance your nervous system and rehydrate connective tissue throughout the body. The techniques offer a way to address the true cause of pain and bring about natural pain relief, rather than masking the symptoms.

The workshop was my first real exposure to words such as fascia, myofascial release, and connective tissue as they relate to pain and the human body. I had heard of rolling your body on very firm foam rollers, and rolling your foot on a lacrosse ball, but didn't know much about either. What little exposure I'd had to rolling was not pleasant, and I'd immediately rejected it.

I entered the workshop dubious. *Besides,* I silently objected, *I wasn't in any physical pain that I was aware of, anyway.* In the workshop, we did a MELT foot treatment. MAN, my feet had not felt that good in a long time! I had had plantar fasciitis several years prior and thought I had totally rehabilitated it at the time. Turns out that it was kind of back, but I had just been tuning it out.

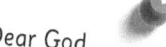

Dear God,

Please help me keep an open mind to things that may help me live more fully in the present. Help me be open to new things I know nothing about. Help me be humble and to give myself permission NOT to be an expert on something. Imagine that.

Since that initial workshop, I have attended three progressive levels of MELT instructor trainings and use the MELT Method both personally and professionally on a regular basis. Thank goodness I listened to my friend and attended that workshop against my better judgment.

# 137
## Another CV/CV Writing Exercise

*My Critical Voice:*
*Dear Sally,*
*Loser, you're huge. You've got the basketball as big as that woman you saw at the grocery store today. You've "failed" menopause. You've failed your son. You've failed your friends. You've got a whole month till the workshop and nothing to do but sit in uncomfortable feelings. As if you could write the Basketball book – You've Got One! Hah!*

*My Compassionate Voice:*
*Dear Sally-Girl,*
*I love you no matter what you eat, even that 4-inch square slab of slightly underdone brownie. I love you no matter what you weigh. I love you ... Basketball stomach or not ... ALWAYS ... period.*

*You can still write the book with a Basketball stomach. Maybe that's part of the journey ... not to avoid it, but to embrace it. Maybe you needed to pad your food tonight to be able to embrace all your sadness over your son growing up. You won't need that much food everyday if you lean into the sadness. You're not a loser. You've failed at nothing and you've failed no one. Failure would mean isolating and NOT sharing this process with other women. That's not you at all.*

*I know a month before your workshop seems an unbelievably long time to wait, but maybe you need this time to process reality. Bottom line: God is here with you. God is going to guide you about MELT Method and your joints; guide you on your food; and guide you in surviving your son growing up. All of it is in God's hands so have an amazing sleep.*

*Now focus on relaxing your tense, knotted upper back.*

*Always remember, God loves you so much He can't take His eyes off you!*

# 138

## "Dear God, I Feel ... Because ...."

*I feel so sad I might die.* My son starts high school tomorrow. That means, in like five minutes, he will be going away to college. Everyone else seems so nonchalant about it, while I'm crying about it. A part of my heart is dying ... literally. He's my baby ... my one and only. This is it. No more babies. No more children. It's over. So sad.

Reflections:
Just for today, I will show up for the full gamut of life. I will feel and express my feelings to another safe human being, and I will also show up for work and use my brain. Even though I would rather stay curled up in a ball in my bed with the shutters closed, I commit to fake it till I make it by showing up for work, trusting that these feelings will pass. The less I pad my food about it, the sooner the feelings will pass. And the less I pad my food about it, the more present I can be for my son, who still needs me very much.

For today I can stay resolute by eating an extra serving of veggies and consuming one less serving of non-nutritional food. Gentle, gentle; perfectly imperfect.

# 139
## My Own Private Summer

*My friend Cordelia* (40) recently experienced dizziness and a racing heart and was sure she was about to faint, or have a heart attack, or both. She'd secretly been vaping tobacco, but she was so freaked out she quit instantly! She'd never experienced anything like it in her life. At the time, she was on a getaway weekend with her boyfriend that ended abruptly with a trip to the ER. Not able to pinpoint the exact nature of her symptoms, the doctor suspended her driver's license with orders to return home and immediately see a cardiologist for further testing. Once at the cardiologist (driven there by her mother), all tests revealed a totally healthy heart. Somewhat puzzled, the doctor asked her to describe what she'd experienced in as much detail as possible. "Well…I felt dizzy, my heart raced, and it was like I was burning up from heat, but the heat was somehow coming from the inside of me…." At hearing this, her mother excitedly jumped up and exclaimed, "That sounds like a HOT FLASH!" Mystery solved.

> Dear Big Love,
> This perimenopause is not for babies. It is real. Please help me find other like-minded, supportive women to surround myself with as I embrace and navigate this uncharted territory.

# 140
## Heat Survival Guide

*It's summer now.* It's bad enough when it's winter because I'm pretty much always experiencing my own private summer on the inside. In my younger days, I was constantly cold. Those days are gone. Now I am always at least warm. When the actual summer season and my internal summer season collide, it is HELL. My hair starts to frizz. My makeup runs. I feel unattractive and uncomfortable, to say the least. And all this can happen just while applying makeup for the day! I keep a small oscillating fan on myself in the bathroom. A thing such as returning to my hot car in a parking lot is akin to a death sentence. It is a thing to be avoided at all costs. I will park and walk extremely long distances to at least be able to park in the shade or in a covered parking structure. This is SERIOUS. Ask my teenaged son. I always carry the LARGEST ice-filled water bottle with me. This is more important than my cell phone. I also keep a monster-sized ice chest in my car with a bag of ice in it from May to October. Sometimes I don't use it for anything; it just helps with my fear of overheating. The last two days in a row I've taken a cold bath in the afternoon.

> Reflections:
>
> Just for today, there are solutions. I can use a fan while I get ready for work this morning. I can carry a large ice water with me wherever I go. I can park in the shade. And I can take a cold shower or bath after work.

# 141

## Shhhhh!!!!

*It's 9:46 p.m.* It's 77 degrees out, with 61 percent humidity. I just met with my friend Cordelia to have a financial lesson: equity, life insurance, 401K, IRA, variable annuity. Yuck. But I digress. For me, the hormonal fluctuation of menopause has brought on my noise aversion. I didn't know there was such a thing, and that it could be associated with menopause. But there is. All kinds of sounds really bug me. For example, when driving, I must have all the windows completely rolled up. If anyone cracks a window, the resulting sound is physically painful. When my husband watches any TV shows that involve gunfire, explosions, or yelling (therefore, anything he watches), it is super annoying. He has gotten headphones. Bless him. I cannot be in a mall food court for long without it becoming annoying. One of our dogs barks incessantly at mealtime and it makes me crazy. Even when the dogs drink water from their water dish, it wakes me up at night. Wait, I'm crossing over into how menopause affects my ability to fall asleep/stay asleep/go back to sleep. That'll be covered another day.

So anyway, it's been hot at night lately. We sleep with the windows open. But our neighbors have been using their air conditioners. Because of my noise aversion issues, I can't go to sleep hearing their A/C, so I close the windows and turn on our A/C. But then the sound of our A/C keeps me awake. So, I turn off the A/C. Now I'm super-hot. Tonight is a lose-lose-lose: Too hot – too much noise – insomnia.

Now WAIT … have I mentioned getting up three or more times per night to urinate? That will also be covered another day!

> Reflections:
> I am going to accept where I am today. And I am going to let my new meditation app help me to go to sleep and stay asleep tonight.

# 142

## Unload the Dishwasher and Move Your Body

*This morning when I awoke,* I felt down immediately ... almost paralyzed. There was nothing "shiny" to look forward to. I hadn't gotten enough sleep the night before either. That made it even more challenging to start the day. I contemplated calling in sick to work. It would've been okay. Besides, I had a challenging client coming to see me today. I decided to pray for guidance and unload the dishwasher while I waited for clarity. Once I'd completed that task, I decided to move my body. Not an epic, Olympic-caliber workout – just move my body. I took a 17-minute bike ride. That's it. I can't tell you how much that helped. Then I was inspired to Swiffer the entryway. I felt even better. Not only did I go to work, I had a fantastic day at work, AND even the challenging client was awesome to work with.

> Dear God,
> Please just get me to the dishwasher so I can connect with You today. Please use me in a powerful way. Thank You!

# 143
## MORE ON UNSCHEDULED, UNCONTROLLABLE CRYING

*My friend Cordelia* (48) arrived at her 12:30 MRI appointment at 12:25. Only problem was it was the kind of appointment where 12:30 really means 12:15 because you must fill out a pile of forms beforehand. The office personnel held the line on the policy and insisted she reschedule. In tears, she tried in vain to explain she was fast at completing forms. She erupted in a tear-filled meltdown as she stormed out of the building. Imagine her discomfort when she returned to her rescheduled appointment later that day to face the same office personnel she had melted down to earlier. Sometimes we just can't control those tears.

Besides going through this myself more than once, I am seeing this more and more in friends of mine. In another case where a group of girlfriends routinely gets together, my friend Cordelia (52) was there as usual. In walked another friend, who rarely meets with us. At the sight of this other friend, without even speaking, Cordelia just burst into tears and sobbed on and off for the next 30 minutes, not sure why. I knew why.

Another friend (51) gets teary all the time while we're chatting on the phone. She'll be talking and suddenly say, "I don't even know why this is making me cry."

I know why. I'll wait till she brings up the Pause, as this can be a touchy subject. At least it was for me.

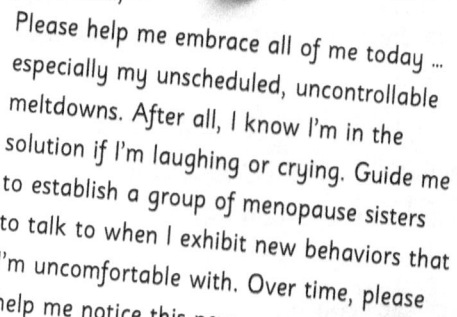

Dear God,
Please help me embrace all of me today ... especially my unscheduled, uncontrollable meltdowns. After all, I know I'm in the solution if I'm laughing or crying. Guide me to establish a group of menopause sisters to talk to when I exhibit new behaviors that I'm uncomfortable with. Over time, please help me notice this new me without judgment.
Make me a channel of Your peace for my menopausal sisters.

# 144

## Maximum Time in a Bra and Bra Replacement Trials

*It's morning.* I put on my "good" bra. It's the one that looks sensational on. It's also the one that I can only stand to wear for about two hours before it starts digging into my back and makes me turn into Linda Blair in *The Exorcist*. After that, it MUST come off. But then the girls don't look quite as sensational. But for some reason, I have found that even if I take say a two-hour break from wearing the "good" bra, and then try to wear it again, it just does not work. It's as if somehow my whole body expands and drops from 3:00 p.m. onward every day, no matter how healthfully I eat, no matter how much water I drink and vegetables

> Dear God,
> For today, help me to remember I am more than my body. Help me to let go of my "impression management" and accept myself and my body as is. Help me to let go of what others think of me.

I consume. There is just NO way I am putting that bra on again today. Every cell of my body protests ... no matter what! Then I switch over to the "kinda" bra. It offers way less support, but it is way more comfortable. It's better than nothing. But I really miss the look of the "good" bra.

# 145
## Just Smell Good

*Let's face it.* Somedays I just feel old. My skin doesn't look the same as it used to. It's looser. My hair doesn't look the same as it once did. It's thinner and graying. Some days, looking at my face in the mirror is pretty discouraging. Then there are the armpits. Do fluctuating hormones affect even body odor? I don't EVER remember smelling this bad. And it's not just the armpits. Those are the days I just say to myself, "Well, at least I can change how I smell!"

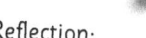

Reflection:
For today, I can take a shower and smell better! I might even take two showers. What a difference it makes! It's the little things.

# 146
## How Many Recipes Can I Turn Green?

*Since childhood,* I have always loved to bake anything sweet. I'm good at it. In my family, I got a lot of attention for my baking skills. I ate most of what I baked, and it was excessive. Over time I came to terms with my eating habits and found peace and solution in a self-help group. Part of my embracing the Pause has been to be more conscious of what I'm eating. Most days, I choose self-loving, nutritious foods and amounts. I've bumped up my vegetable consumption. Some people spend a lot of time focusing on what NOT to eat. As a former volume-eater, I want to focus on what TO eat such as vegetables. I've done a lot of experimenting with ways to add more of them in fun ways.

I eat nutritiously about 75 percent of the time. It's boring. But I feel GREAT! For years, I thought eating right was about maintaining my weight. But with the advent of the Pause, I have a whole new angle. When I make self-loving food choices, my eyes look way less puffy in the morning, and so does my stomach. My "good" Bra feels less restricting. My clothes fit better. Even wrinkles on my knees look better. I can MOVE more easily! However, sometimes I just want something sweet and I have found that adding vegetables helps combat some of the above symptoms. Here are two suggestions:

- Add 1-2 cups grated carrots/zucchini to carrot cake mix and substitute baby food prunes for half the oil. Skip the frosting.
- Add 1-2 cups grated zucchini to chocolate cake mix and substitute half the oil with baby food prunes or canned pumpkin. Again, skip the frosting.

The cookbook *Forks over Knives* has several great fruit smoothie recipes with kale and spinach added.

Sometimes I just want a milkshake. I want to hold that cup and drink from a straw like a normal person! I make a milkshake using one percent milk and add kale/spinach, salted caramel frozen yogurt, a squeeze of chocolate syrup, 1Tb. peanut butter and ice.

> Dear God,
> Please give me the willingness to choose self-loving foods and amounts today.

# 147

## Friends Don't Let PM Friends "Suck It Up, Buttercup!"

*I've talked myself out of writing this book again* for about a week now. The critical voice in my head said, "Who are you to think you are an expert on this?"

I met my friend Cordelia (45) for dinner tonight. We'd not gotten together for over a month. It felt good to catch each other up on our lives. We were about to leave the restaurant when she casually mentioned she broke down crying to her husband recently. She told him he needed to take away her sleeping aids because she was concerned she'd overdose on them. As in—she was that depressed. She went on, "… the kids don't need me anymore and I won't live as an invalid."

I questioned her: "Wait, are you saying you're worried you'll commit suicide because you're so depressed?" She nodded. Then I heard My Compassionate Voice whispering to me again, saying, "You've got to write the book! Cordelia and so many others need the book!"

My book is on again. "Cordelia," I said, "it's menopause! You're gonna be okay!" She said she'd been exercising and eating healthier, but she'd gained 20 pounds and was so frustrated. Of course she was! Menopause! She continued on about the sweating, the new and incredibly offensive body odor, the crying, along with an "everything-is-the-end-of-the-world" attitude. I told her about Omega 3 fish oil and my 24/7 giant ice water cup glued to my hip. The book is SO back on. "Why didn't you call me sooner?" I asked. "Because my mom always says, Suck it up, buttercup!"

Reflections:
Cordelia, don't suck it up, buttercup! Not this time. Talk about it with your girlfriends! You are NOT alone. Your life is SO not over! And I need to persevere, following my heart and believing in myself.

# 148
## Physical Pain/Aging

*Okay*, I wanted a way to connect with my preteen son, so at 52 years of age, I joined his taekwon-do class. That shouldn't have been a problem, right? Three years, many side splits, roundhouse kicks, movement pattern memorizations, sparring matches, and a variety of board breaks later, I proudly received my 1st degree black belt alongside my son, who was receiving his 2nd degree black belt simultaneously. It was an enormous undertaking for a woman in her 50s and I don't regret it for an instant. The resulting bond with my son is worth every struggle I encountered along the way.

However, what I failed to take into consideration was that I was in a 50 plus-year-old newly menopausal body with no prior martial arts experience. The movement pattern memorization alone nearly killed me! But don't you know who I am? I can do anything I set my mind to. And I did. But there were consequences. One of which was physical pain: pain in my hip and thigh. I attended exactly one class wearing my beautiful, stiff new black belt and told the Master I would need to take some time off. I assumed my hip pain would stop as soon as I discontinued my practice.

I went 10 months without practicing taekwon-do. My pain continued. I tried stretching, massages, multiple physical therapists, and acupuncture, to name a few. No one could even give me a concrete diagnosis. The pain got worse at times. I got x-rays and MRIs of both my hip and my lumbar spine. I went to a prominent hip surgeon who said I did not need a hip replacement. He gave me a cortisone shot. I was pain-free for about a week. The pain returned. The pain worsened. I began to limp.

Dear God,
Sometimes things take a long time to heal, a REALLY long time ... much longer than I expect. And it may require a combination of solutions. Help me to trust You and turn to You in all situations for my solutions. Help me to believe there IS a solution. Help me not to become discouraged and to keep seeking solutions, even when I think I have already tried every possible solution.

# 149
## Don't Quit Before the Miracle

*By the time my mystery pain* had dragged on for approximately three years (2012–2014), I was beside myself with frustration. Two physical therapists, a chiropractor, and a prominent orthopedic hip surgeon could not diagnose the cause of my hip and thigh pain. I used pain pills with limited success. I soon ruled them out due to unacceptable risks and side effects.

One afternoon I cried in the grocery store parking lot because I could barely walk from my car to the store without stopping several times to rest. Don't you know I am a fitness instructor? It's especially important that I be able to walk! I can't be limping! My then-teenaged son later told me he had watched me in horror from the car, not sure what was wrong with me. At that point I was desperate for a solution. I sensed the MELT method could help me, but was unsure exactly how to use it for that purpose. Even though I had had beginning MELT Method training, I felt I needed more training. Meanwhile, my pain continued. I attended a second MELT Method training (summer 2014).

Since the creator of MELT, Sue Hitzmann and I live on opposite coasts, I sought a local MELT instructor to help me hone my newly-acquired MELT teaching skills. Through networking at my MELT Method training, I got the name of an experienced MELT instructor who also just happened to be a myofascial release therapist and was also completing her doctorate in physical therapy. After over a year of a combination of myofascial release and MELT Method self-treatment techniques, I was able to walk without a limp. I began to see light at the end of the tunnel.

> Dear God,
> Sometimes I just want to give up and take painkillers for the rest of my life. Please help me to believe there is ALWAYS a solution that includes staying in the present.

The road back to being pain-free has been long. It began with swimming with only my arms. No legs. No strength training. Besides swimming with arms only, I could use the arm bike. That's all. I am PM! Don't you know exercise is one of my PM antidrugs?! Did I mention I work in fitness?

Don't you know I need those endorphins? Never in my worst nightmare could I have predicted how slow the recovery would be. Although I have been down at times, I have never given up hope.

> **Call to Action:**
> Think about something you are feeling discouraged about, or have given up on. Are you willing to open your mind to new solutions?

# 150

## THERE MAY BE SETBACKS ... DON'T GIVE UP

*Today my leg was hurting.* Two days ago, it felt the best it's felt in months. I was so excited; I swam four laps using my legs. It didn't hurt at all! Today it hurt most of the day. I'm so disappointed. Tonight, we're having Mexican food at a favorite restaurant. I'd like to eat a basket of chips and salsa. I deserve it.

Reflections:
For Today, I'll get into the solution. The way out of a negative feeling is a positive decision followed by action. Just as we left the table, I grabbed two chips and ate them. The good news is that there were a lot of chips remaining in the basket. Also, I spent ten minutes on my soft foam roller. My body feels a lot better and so does my mind and spirit.

# 151

## Annual Female Checkup

*Today was my annual female checkup.* My OB/Gyn recommended I try a new procedure she offers called Mona Lisa Touch. Mona Lisa Touch is a laser treatment for vaginal rejuvenation that gives effective relief and offers life-changing results for women. It has been clinically proven to provide effective results for vaginal dryness, vaginal laxity, and mild urinary incontinence. It was a strange sensation but not at all painful.

> Dear God,
> I know I am always striving to be open to new things, but even under the hood? What next?

# 152

## Hot Yoga & the Shortest Route to Insanity

I visited my friend Cordelia (45) recently. She has fallen in love with hot yoga. She insisted I join her. Always a competitor, even when someone is 10 years my junior, I acquiesced. Oh, did I mention she does hot yoga in a bikini? And her body is perfect? I think yoga is a wonderful thing, but it is not really my thing. After 90 minutes of hot yoga situated directly behind my bikini'd friend, it took me over 48 hours to reset my brutal negative self-talk. Just the "hot" alone could have been a clue for me to politely decline. Live and learn. How nice am I that I wanted to do what my friend loves without concern for what is best for me?

> Dear God,
> Help me remember that comparison is the shortest route to insanity.

# 153

## Channel Your PM Energy in a Positive Way

*My friend Cordelia* (56) is showing signs of PM. As is usually the case, I recognize PM signs in others long before they realize them in themselves. Yesterday she came home from work early … 2:00 p.m. She ate three doughnuts and a bag of chips and went straight to bed and basically slept through the night. Today she began her period for the second time in four weeks.

During the day today, she received one of those IRS scam voicemail messages on her phone, insisting she must "call this number immediately" to avoid further charges because she was being audited by the IRS. I've received those types of scam voicemails many times. So has she. She has usually just ignored them but not today. Today, she called the number back. A live person answered. She could tell it was a cell phone she was calling. She told the man he was full of it and that she was going to report him. The man challenged her. "If you don't believe me, why are you still on the phone?" he asked. "… because … I AM COMING FOR YOU!" she half-screamed. He hung up on her. She wasn't satisfied. Next, she posted his number on the IRS fraud website.

Cordelia wasn't done. She THEN posted his number on her Facebook account and asked her friends to join her in text-bombing the guy. Last I heard, she plans to send him texts every time she thinks of it until the feelings pass. Way to turn things around!

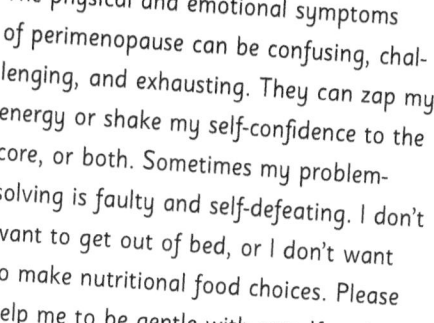

Dear God,

The physical and emotional symptoms of perimenopause can be confusing, challenging, and exhausting. They can zap my energy or shake my self-confidence to the core, or both. Sometimes my problem-solving is faulty and self-defeating. I don't want to get out of bed, or I don't want to make nutritional food choices. Please help me to be gentle with myself and to channel my PM energy in a positive and humorous and powerful way … the way Cordelia did.

# 154
## And Then There's the Issue of Memory

*Wednesday:* I was working with clients and was inspired about an exercise I wanted to have them to do. It was exactly right for them and I was excited about it. But just as quickly as the idea came into my brain, it departed.

Friday at bedtime: The exercise came back to me! Oh well, I'll see them again in a week. Better luck next time.

Other times while working, I will excitedly come up with two great exercises simultaneously. Invariably, my brain becomes instantaneously overloaded by this and I simply cannot remember either idea.

> Dear God,
> Help me to be gentle with myself when my brain and memory aren't what they used to be.

# 155
## Mentally Preparing:
## Humility Without Judgment and Letting Go of the Results

*As cliché as it may sound,* I've spent years learning to be "me" and be okay with that. Nevertheless, in some situations in life, it behooves me to edit the Full Monty Sally Bartlett, if you will. Yesterday I had an appointment with an attorney about a real estate issue. Meeting with attorneys is not something I do on a regular basis. It is extremely uncomfortable for me because in the past, it has led to conversations where I do not understand the jargon being used and do not know answers to questions I am asked that lead to shame and feeling stupid. I pride myself on being intelligent and when I don't understand something I can immediately jump to unworthiness. Knowing this about myself, I mentally prepared myself before the appointment.

She may ask a question I don't know the answer to.

Even though I'm as prepared as I can possibly be, she may need paperwork other than what I've brought.

She's not my girlfriend. Stay on topic. The clock is ticking. No chitchat.

After the appointment, I was elated. I did it! I calmly, nonjudgmentally answered, "I don't know" when I didn't. The attorney didn't laugh me out of her office. She didn't announce on the office loudspeaker: "Hey, everyone! Get this: Sally Bartlett doesn't know what this means!" She even asked me a question about what I do for a living and I answered, but quickly and seamlessly returned to the topic on hand. I left her office walking tall!

Once back in my car, I realized I needed to "thaw out" from my hyper-professional demeanor. To help myself relax and breathe a little, I started calling girlfriends, bookending how things had gone at the appointment. It took a good hour to return to my normal semi-carefree state. All things considered, I'd say that's fast.

Some days I just need to be me and embrace that. Other days call for a mental pep talk so that my expectations are appropriate to the situation. With the help of the Universe, I can do this.

> Dear God,
> Please guide me in Your will for me today. Use me in a powerful way.

# 156
## Feeling Vulnerable, Tender and Fragile

*The morning after the appointment with the attorney,* I happened to have scheduled my annual mammogram, which this year included both abdominal and pelvic ultrasounds. At the time, I thought nothing about the fact that one day I would be doing really super grown-up things and the next day I would be mostly naked while having various body parts poked and squished in super-compromising positions … while menopausal … on an empty stomach … with a full bladder.

About two hours later, I emerged from the imaging office, ready to eat an entire tray of pastries. I had the day off and a full list of things I'd planned to accomplish before picking up my son from school. It didn't go quite as planned. I ended up staying in sweats the rest of the day, lacking the energy or desire to apply makeup or shower. I was lucky to have the energy to comb my hair, albeit half-heartedly. What was wrong with me? I fancy myself as a very efficient person. This level of achievement was subpar for me. After writing down my thoughts, I realized the back-to-back events of these two consecutive days had left me feeling vulnerable, fragile, and tender. Despite my ambitious to-do list for today, I sat on the couch and watched the *American Idol* finale over again instead.

> Dear God,
>
> Help me to remember that feelings are not facts. They will pass. Even though I may feel vulnerable, fragile, and tender, it doesn't mean I am those things. I am also safe, strong, and tenacious. Help me to embrace Your perfect balancing of both sides of my emotions.

# 157
## Hot Seat

*We're on the second week of a heat wave.* And it's humid. I cannot cool off. Today I swam laps in hopes of cooling off, but I was even hot in the freakin' pool. The other day while driving, that familiar burning hot feeling came over me that grew and grew. It felt so hot it felt as if my seat warmer was on!

Oh. Turns out it WAS on. I'd accidentally bumped it on with my purse upon entering the car. BUT never mind that. I truly feel "seat-warmer-hot" most of the time these days even when there's no seat warmer turned on. When I'm this warm, I'm about to break into a sweat. When I break into a sweat, I perspire all over, my hair frizzes and looks lame, and I feel like my whole body starts to kinda melt and expand. In short, I feel gross and unattractive, so why not just eat a Costco hotdog, which means a ton of salt, and the whole chain reaction worsens and repeats!

> Reflections:
> Just for today I can:
> • Carry my gigantic ice water with me at all times
> • Take a(nother) cold bath
> • Stock up on veggies

# 158

## DEPRESSION

*Some days I feel blue.* I feel sad. Today was one of those days. It's Sunday. I stayed in bed till 10:00 a.m. There's nothing wrong with that, but I'm typically up by 8:00 a.m. at the latest and off to the gym. Today the solution was to go with what my body was telling me. Eventually (12:45 p.m.) I got to the gym and did a very abbreviated version of my workout and let that be okay. Then I lovingly dragged myself to the grocery store to buy ingredients for my favorite raw zucchini salad recipe. I lovingly coaxed myself to prepare and eat it.

Some days are just like that. I don't need to make it worse by making non-nutritional food choices. Tomorrow's a new day. Trust the (hormonal) process.

- Make/keep self-loving food contract
- 15-minute declutter
- QuickBooks

- Cold bath
- Watch TV dance competition show *So You Think You Can Dance* (again)
- Load dishwasher
- Write a letter to God and have God write me back

*Letter to God:*
*Dear God,*
*Today I feel depressed. I felt down all day. I feel so sad because [fill in the blank]. What will the future hold? How will I ever survive?*
*Love, Sally*

*Letter from God to me:*
*Dear Sally,*
*I love how you stayed in bed today till 10:00 a.m.! I love how you got to the gym eventually anyway. I love how you got the ingredients, prepared, and ate cold zucchini salad. Trust in yourself and take it one day at a time. Always remember, I love you so much I can't take My eyes off you.*
*Love, God*

# 159
## Mother/Son Moment

*The other day* my teenaged son and I were sitting in the car talking and he gazed at me with loving eyes as he contemplated my face. I felt the love. I was touched. I reveled in this special mother/son moment. Then he goes, "Mom, your eyebrows are so cool. They start near the bridge of your nose and continue out and around to the outside of your forehead … and then they curve around and continue all the way down the side of your face…." OMG! Thank you?

> Dear God,
> Please help me remember not to take myself too seriously.

# 160

## Mediocre Meditation

*It seems like everywhere I go,* people are talking about the importance of meditation … for years now. I've tried it a few times. I couldn't get the hang of the "eyes open" part nor the fact that I needed to sit. I can never get comfortable sitting. One day a friend recommended a meditation app. It offered a free trial. I installed it on my phone. I lay down on my bed and pushed play. It instructed the listener to sit rather than lie down. And I was instructed to begin by breathing deeply with my eyes open.

> Reflection:
> Just do it … even if it's mediocre.

So instead, I remained supine and closed my eyes. I loved it. I am still using the app almost every day, sometimes twice a day, three years later. I'm not doing it perfectly. I'm doing a mediocre job and it's fantastic. I usually fall asleep within one minute of the guy saying, "Hi and welcome to day seven." It doesn't matter. Me compared to me, I'm an amazing meditator!

# 161

## On the Lighter Side

*My son drinks a juice smoothie* almost every day. Often, I call ahead to speed up the process. Today I called and got a busy signal. I tried several more times on the way there with the same result (I can be a little compulsive). Upon arriving at the register, I casually asked the teenaged cashier if the store's phone was off the hook. "Huh?" I repeated myself, and added for clarification, "I kept getting a busy signal." "Huh?" I suddenly realized that given his age, he wouldn't know what "off the hook" or "busy signal" meant! I laughed to myself. Even though he was clueless, he apologized politely and gave me $3 off my drink for whatever inconvenience I was talking about and yelled to his supervisor, "Joanne, the phone's broken!" I smiled

Reflections:
Just for today I can make eye contact and connect with people of all ages. I can also laugh at myself and embrace who I am and the life I have lived and am still living.

and was about to let the supervisor in on my joke with myself when I realized that she was also too young to know about old-school phone jargon. She picked up the phone and looked at it, shrugged and walked off. At least I got a laugh ... and a discount.

# 162

## My Feet Are Hot

*It was early November* in Southern California. When is it going to cool off? I like to say our summers are from August to November. Because of a few foot issues I've had for years, athletic shoes with my custom orthotics are my shoes of choice. They are better than my sandals … and to me, way cuter. The sandals that are comfortable to me are super ugly, so ugly that I feel cuter and more feminine in my athletic shoes than in my sandals.

But no matter how thin my socks or how much foot powder I use, it never fails. By about 3:00 p.m. it starts to feel like I've got hot lava in my shoes. It's extremely uncomfortable. My shoes MUST come off. Fifteen years ago, I discovered that taking fish oil before bed eliminated night sweats. I wonder … if I take fish oil in the morning, will my afternoon foot sweating be eliminated as well?

> Dear God,
> Help me embrace yet another new menopausal development with love and grace.

# 163

## Driver's Ed, Doughnuts & Improved Quality Family Time:
### Part I

*Our son has his driving permit.* Let's just say he is not in a huge hurry to drive. Each Sunday my husband and I accompany him as he practices. My son has chosen me to be in the passenger seat while his father sits in the back seat. I suppose I should feel flattered, but this is a very scary place for me to be! Things can be a little tense, but little by little we are learning what works and what doesn't.

For example, I have learned to talk only about things that affect his immediate driving safety. Sometimes my husband and I get on tangents that only distract our son. Today my husband brought up Uncle Mike's seizure in detail. Our son reminded us of acceptable topics during driving practice. I started a list of what topics we would save to discuss over doughnuts. My husband and I got back on topic. Each of us gives an opinion about how to handle a driving skill, such as staying centered in your lane. Then we let our son decide if he thinks that either suggestion would work for him. In short, this experience has led to the best, most productive and most calm communication our family has ever had! Who knew practice-driving could lead to improved family communication and quality time together?

We end each lesson at the doughnut shop. I normally enjoy a doughnut about once a month on New Wave Day, but I decided to change my routine during the driving experience, at least for the time being. That means each Sunday I enjoy a doughnut as I collect myself, relieved that we all survived. Then I take the wheel and drive us home. Last week, while savoring my doughnut, my son announced he would like to drive some more after doughnuts. This is a huge breakthrough. This meant his confidence was increased! I knew I had to say YES! But this threw me for a loop! I didn't think it possible to subject myself to another of his driving sessions, without knowing a doughnut was waiting at the other end! I reluctantly agreed, secretly fearing my nervous system would completely give out. But it didn't. The drive home was uneventful.

Dear God,
Help us all remember that each driving session is a new, improved experience. We are learning how to better communicate with each other. Help me to remember and acknowledge to my son that he is making so much progress each session. Next week I might be able to trust You enough to have a bagel instead of a doughnut!

# 164

## Driver's Ed, Doughnuts & Improved Quality Family Time: Part II

*Today was the fourth Sunday* we have had Driving and Doughnuts. As we started down a big hill, I silently asked God to be with us and watch over us in this huge, heavy moving metal object, and reminded myself I am not the one in charge. I announced that I would prefer a bagel. After my son successfully parallel-parked and got his doughnuts, we proceeded to the bagel shop before heading home.

Dear God,

Help me to remember that even though I have a responsibility to take appropriate care of my child as his mother, I also have a responsibility to take appropriate care of myself and my body. I can speak up and choose self-loving foods and amounts in every situation, to the best of my ability. Help me to remember and acknowledge to myself that I make so much progress with each driving session. I am flexible and capable of growing and changing to meet each new situation life brings to me.

# 165
## Mother/Son Bonding Over Chin Hairs

I don't know about you, but I think it super weird that both my son and I have chin hairs. My son wishes his would increase and spread. I would be happy if I could transport mine onto his face. Then we would both be happy.

> Dear God,
> What do
> You think?

# 166

## I Expect an Award!

*I work hard at everything I do.* I am intense. Whatever I am undertaking, I am balls-to-the-wall. Consequently, often I feel I "should" get an award for my efforts. I don't know who I expect to receive this award from, but it should happen … maybe my friends or my husband. I deem all sorts of accomplishments "award-worthy," big or small. If I complete an amazing day at work, I want an award. I want an award if I make my bed (including all the pillows). Somedays I want an award for putting on makeup. I want an award for washing my hair. I want an award for replacing a light bulb. I want an award for … you get the idea. If no one comes forward to give me my expected award, I tend to want to reward myself with non-nutritional food.

> Call to Action:
> List one way you can award yourself besides overeating.

> Dear God,
> Please help me not to be so dependent on external validation.
> Just for Today I can give myself an award. I can make myself nutritional treats and freeze ahead to have handy. I can take myself out for an iced tea. I can take a bath and put lotion on my feet before bed.

# 167

## THY WILL BE DONE

*Dear God,*
*What is Your will for me on this book? Now that I have read it all, I realize I wrote the bulk of material in the early awareness about my perimenopausal journey. Then I wrote about 10 percent more later in my journal. That seems disjointed. I just want to scrap the whole thing because I pictured it unfolding in a certain way, and that's not what happened. Is it still valuable and if so, how? Has this just been a nice reminder exercise for me to have revisited my journey, period? I am called to share this with the world. Is that what You are telling me? If so, how do I accomplish that? Or is this nothing more than my "personal agenda" to have external validation? Oh, and do I include my recipes? Please advise!*
*Love, Sally*

*Dear Sally-Girl,*

*I keep gently telling you, "Just follow your inner voice. Listen to the voice that keeps saying 'someone needs to hear your message.' Don't worry about continuity. Just write. Just put one foot in front of the other. Easy does it ... one step at a time. Just do it. Let go of your mental picture of how things 'should' unfold. Answers will come."*
*Love, God*

> Call to Action:
> If there is still that small voice urging you to do something, listen to it.

# 168

## Depression Spiral

*I have the day off.* It always surprises me, but sometimes days off are the hardest days for me. There is so much I hope to accomplish. I want to work on the book. It is 9:48 a.m., and I haven't even showered. I have been home for one hour, puttering around the house doing minutiae. I cannot seem to get myself into the shower. Every time I say to myself "Time to shower," I can't decide if I should wash my hair or not, and I get stuck there. I feel so much better when I do, but it takes so long. Still undecided, I go try to pump up my BOSU instead. BOSU is an acronym for Both Sides Up or Both Sides Utilized. This wonderful prop is a fitness and balance training tool, consisting of an inflated rubber dome attached to a rigid platform. Performing an ordinary squat while standing atop the rounded edge of the BOSU increases both the athletic difficulty and the result exponentially. Highly recommend!  Attention Deficit Disorder much?

Anyway, my BOSU pump doesn't work, so I go up to my computer and check on Amazon for a pump adapter and order one. Then again, I ask myself, "Should I wash my hair or not?" And so it goes for about an hour. Finally, I just decide to wash my hair because it's easier than trying to figure out if my hair looks okay without washing it today. Now I only must decide what to wear ….

> Reflection:
> I bought myself flowers.
> Some days are like that
> … gentle, gentle.

# 169

## Human-Doing

*It's 6:00 p.m. I am tired.* I've put in a full day of administrative to-dos, motherhood duties, and the like. My to-do list is not nearly completed. I could use a short nap before resuming the evening's motherhood duties that includes driving to martial arts. Don't get me wrong. I LOVE being a mom and spending any time my son wants to spend with me. Nevertheless, I am so tired that even my necklace seems to have gotten heavier on my neck and has become a burden. If I can just squeeze in one more thing….

> Call to Action:
> Get yourself in a supine position and stay there for 15 minutes, with your shoes off.

No, wait! I think I could stay in the present better if I stopped what I am doing and got horizontal with my shoes removed. I need to remind myself to strive to be a Human

Being instead of a Human-Doing. There is time to stop and get horizontal ... with shoes off. Even if just for 15 minutes. Really, I'm going to try it.

15 minutes later ... and I'm back to my writing. I made a contract with myself to get horizontal, without shoes, and I kept it. It feels indescribably wonderful.

# 170

## Reset Button for Expectations

*This time,* before visiting my bikini-donning yoga friend, I mentally prepared by reminding myself:

She's 10 years younger than I am.

Her house is 7,000 square feet and mine is … not.

The exercise journey in me honors the exercise journey in her.

She is a very sophisticated dresser 24/7.

I wore my jeans and a T-shirt and my long-drive bra.

They drink alcohol. I don't.

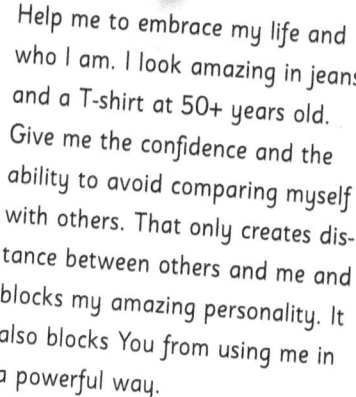

Dear God,
Help me to embrace my life and who I am. I look amazing in jeans and a T-shirt at 50+ years old. Give me the confidence and the ability to avoid comparing myself with others. That only creates distance between others and me and blocks my amazing personality. It also blocks You from using me in a powerful way.

Help me remember comparison is the shortest route to insanity.

# 171
## Asking for What I Want

*Dear God,*
*I feel like eating because I said what was on my mind today and asked for what I want. I'm worried I pissed off at least two people and one institution.*

*Dear Sally-Girl,*
*I know it feels like you'll die from people being mad at you. But you won't. You took care of yourself. You calmly, appropriately said how you felt and/or asked for what you wanted. Way to go! Great job! Continue to have the courage to ask for what you want. Award!*
*Love, God*

# 172

## DISCIPLINE LEADS TO HAPPINESS; SPONTANEITY LEADS TO CHAOS

*My friend Cordelia* (65) commented to me that she was frustrated. She kept making non-nutritive food choices and as a result, her weight wasn't where she wanted it to be. I sympathized with her. I reminded her I have maintained a 35-lb. weight loss for over 30 years. I know how hard it can be to continue to choose self-loving foods and amounts meal after meal … day after day, year after year. Just as I have learned to do with my teenager, I asked whether she just wanted me to listen, or if she wanted suggestions. She wanted suggestions. I asked her for an example of what she is frustrated about. And she shared, "Yesterday I went out to breakfast with friends and I chose a waffle. I felt terrible both physically and mentally as I walked from the restaurant. And my non-nutritious choices at breakfast set the tone for my food choices for the rest of my day."

I really relate to her example. I've come to learn to ask friends for help on these types of food-centered social occasions. When I encounter this situation, I use a tool called bookending. Years ago, a wise woman taught me to call someone before a situation to bookend—or be accountable—with my food commitment. Afterward, I call back with the second bookend about whether I kept my commitment. If I don't keep the commitment I made, it isn't a reason to beat myself up. It means I made my commitment too difficult to keep and to make it easier or less stringent next time.

Additionally, and especially during the holiday season, I can make a commitment to myself and another understanding person that I will make one new huge nutritious, veggie-laden recipe once every two weeks. An added bonus: I can freeze the extra for future use.

Dear God,

Help me remember that social situations are about the people, not the food. The more I can stay present with the people I'm with, the more I connect with them. I can look up most restaurants online ahead of time and bookend with a trusted friend before and after I eat. Please empower me!

Taking these small actions makes me feel very loved and cared for ... by me! By doing this, I take responsibility for my own health and sense of well-being. Over time, it adds up exponentially. It's empowering and uplifting! Dr. Patricia Allen writes:

*Discipline leads to happiness; Spontaneity leads to chaos. I know how much I love myself by the contracts I'm willing to make and keep.*

# 173

## WHAT AM I LOOKING FORWARD TO TODAY?

*My friend Cordelia* commented to me that while she loves her huge family and spending time with them, she didn't feel as though she was getting time to do things she really enjoyed doing. By the time she got done doing for everyone else, there was simply no time left for herself and the things that make her heart sing, like sewing. We talked about the possibility of her taking responsibility for own happiness each day.

Reflections:
Help me remember to consider what I am looking forward to today. Please give me the willingness to plan something into my day for me ... even if just for 15 minutes.

# 174
## The Power of Music

*I'm at the gym* on the elliptical with *Beautiful: The Carole King Musical* playing on my headphones. The overture has barely begun to play and I am in tears. I don't even fully understand why I'm in tears; I just know it's a good thing and I let it happen. It had something to do with my teenage years and remembering how much I was moved by her music so long ago. Music can be so healing. I try to wipe my tears as inconspicuously as possible. But I realize I don't really care all that much what I may look like. I just feel good.

Meanwhile, the guy in front of me on the bike is that guy that's always at the gym. He is so into his music that he is practically dancing off the seat with his upper body, including his own unique style of hairology. It is quite a spectacle. It borders on crazy when he seems to conduct a symphony at certain parts. In between enjoying my tears and my rising endorphin level, I wonder if his over-the-top-head-shaking to the beat-of-his-music-sweat-dripping head may spray sweat onto me. The thought momentarily grosses me out. Luckily, I am just out of reach, thank You, God. I smile and laugh to myself. My music continues to move me to still more tears. Another man walks by and I watch him watch the über-sweaty rocking-out guy and shake his head and smile. I smile and cry simultaneously. I feel so good.

> Dear God,
> Life is always ebbing and flowing. Help me be in the moment and enjoy this "flowing" experience. Thank You!

# 175
# Hormone Replacement Therapy Journey

*I am 60 years of age* as I write this entry and have not had a menstrual cycle since age 50. I consider myself menopausal. Looking back on this journey, I have gracefully (eventually) come to terms with and embraced The Pause. I currently see the original OB/Gyn doctor I first saw when this journey began around age 45. Not too long after beginning this journey with her, she moved her practice to a town about two hours away from where I lived. I considered continuing to see her, but decided the drive was too much.

For a short period of time, I tried many other doctors. None was anywhere near as knowledgeable and helpful as my original doctor. She gets peri- and menopause. She gets me. Several months and seven doctors later, I decided two hours wasn't such a long drive after all. I have happily made the trek once a year for over nine years.

Also over a period of about 15 years, I tried several different medications, including two different types of oral birth control, an antidepressant, two types of bioidentical hormone patches, two sleep aids, an estradiol vaginal ring, and custom blend hormone cream from a compound pharmacy.

Part of it was trial-and-error under my doctor's supervision, seeing what helped and what didn't. But on top of that, my hormones constantly fluctuated, making it necessary to change meds yet again. To keep abreast of hormone levels, I have had lab work done twice per year through all of this. Some years (depending on how good my medical insurance was that year) I have also done a 24-hour urine collection. This is super tedious and complicated, and practically requires you to be a rocket scientist to complete. But evidently it results in the most accurate hormone levels.

So, what's the upshot of all this? With the help of a few OTC supplements, I am feeling so much better these days. Currently, and for the past year, the only prescription I take is the custom blended hormone cream and the very occasional quarter of a sleep aid. I continue to take OTC supplements wherever my lab work indicates vitamin deficiencies.

Dear God,

Please give me patience with myself during this process. Help me trust I will find the right hormonal balance. Give me strength. Please hurry. I need You.

# 176

## LEARN SOMETHING NEW

*Sometimes* I get into fear of financial insecurity in my head. My head just won't quit. "What are you going to do when your husband retires?" "How will you afford to live?" Recently my head was going crazy with that kind of talk. So much so that I called a girlfriend and expressed this. I didn't like her response. "Well, it sounds like it might be time to learn a new skill."

Learn a new skill? No! Next thing I know I am online looking at the schedule of classes at the local community college. I'm signing up for accounting 1A, a four-unit, transferrable college course. GROSS. Next, thing I know I am attending the first day of this 16-week course at 57 years old with a room full of 18-year-olds.

I understood little of the first lecture. The professor encouraged me to hang in there for the first three chapters before deciding to drop the course. I did. I got a 78 percent on the first exam. But by then I was three chapters into it and even enjoyed class at times. I got a 98 percent on the second exam. I was euphoric.

I really don't even care about the grade. I'm extremely challenged by the class, but the point is, I am learning a lot about money and things I've never understood.

And remember that fear-based voice in my head? It's SO gone!

> Reflection:
> Just for today I can step out of my comfort zone and try something that challenges my brain. Who knows, I may even like it.

# 177
## Where Do I Fit Here?

*Okay,* then there was an accounting class team project and oral presentation. The professor informed us he'd be breaking us into teams of four. I was probably more nervous about breaking into teams than I was about taking an accounting course in the first place. It was one thing to sit quietly in a room taking notes, but to speak to and interact with others around me? What would the other three kids assigned to my group think? Would they be so bummed that they got me in their group? How should I act? What should I wear? I didn't want to embarrass myself by trying to sound or dress too cool. After all, I was basically older than most of their mothers.

The day teams were announced, I continued to take deep breaths as inconspicuously as possible. I lived through it. Sometimes I must remind myself that the rest of the world is just as self-obsessed as I am, so I don't need to worry so much. The group project and presentation came and went, and I lived through that, too. As with most scary things I walk through, a huge sense of accomplishment, pride, and serenity came with completion of the project.

Toward the end of the semester, something happened that put everything into perspective for me. As I walked into the classroom and took my usual seat, one of my fellow students casually said to me, "You finish the homework?" I was reminded at that moment I can do anything. No matter how old I am, I can always fit in if I am willing to sit with temporary discomfort and walk through fear.

The semester was finally over, and I earned an A in the class. But way better than that, I got to walk through a fear, increase accounting knowledge, and increase my self-confidence.

> Dear God,
> Please give me the courage and the willingness to walk through discomfort so that You can use me in a powerful way. It is so worth it.

# 178
## BREAK OUT OF YOUR ROUTINE

*I love routine. I love structure.* I love my Sunday routine. Then one day, Cordelia (48) texted to invite me to go to a craft show near the ocean with her that Sunday. It's a good thing people cannot hear you when they text you. "Oh, NO, I am so not going to that!" For one thing, I didn't know this person very well. Plus, I find some craft shows to be kind of cheesy. I mentally cataloged several reasons NOT to go. What if she loved cheesy craft shows? What if she liked to stay the entire day? What if she eats weird food that's not like the way I eat? Will parking be hard? Do I have to give up my favorite workout for that day? It became a ridiculous case of contempt prior to investigation.

Dear God,
Please help me to let go occasionally. I might even have a good time and make a new friend.

I texted her back and got more information. Against my "better" judgment, I decided to go! I ended up really enjoying spending time with the friend. It turned out we had a lot in common. I had a really good time and I am so glad I stepped out of my comfort zone and broke out of my routine for one day.

# 179
## Green With Envy

*A good friend of mine* just received an amazing job offer for yet another new job. This is probably the third time I have witnessed this happening to her over the years, where, without any action whatsoever on her part, she is presented with a job interview and subsequent job offer, complete with pay increase and career advancement.

Why don't I get lucrative job offers all the time (or freakin' ever) like my friend? I want mine!

- I deserve financial abundance
- I attract financial abundance

Dear God,
Help me to remember when You aren't showering me with obvious amazing good fortune, You are wanting me to grow closer to You instead. And help me to remember that maybe this is a time in my life where You want me to slow down and spend more time with my son before he goes off to college. And that maybe I am right where I am supposed to be right now in this moment. Help me to bloom where I am planted, instead of driving myself crazy by comparing my insides to someone else's outsides.

# 180

## Make a New Green Smoothie

*I love making smoothie drinks* in my blender for breakfast. Basically, they all have greens, plain Greek yogurt, almond milk, ice, and fruit. I change the fruit for variety. I was really into mixed berries for quite a while. But then I got sick of it. I'd done everything I could think of: pineapple and mango with lime; pear and banana with almond butter. But at the craft fair with Cordelia, I discovered green juice that had grapefruit in it. It sounded gross. But I tried it. I didn't like it and made a sour face. But after about 10 seconds, I was craving more of it. I bought it. I became obsessed with making a smoothie with similar ingredients. Hence the greens, grapefruit, apple, pineapple green smoothie was born. I am so excited about it! It's quite refreshing for

> Dear God,
> Thank You for open-mindedness. Thank You for showing me a better use of "Green" besides envy.

the hot days that are coming. Note: this was written before I (imperfectly) let go of dairy (teardrop). BUT the smoothies all taste just as good without the yogurt!

# 181

## The Fitness Journey in Me Honors the Fitness Journey in You

*I played several sports competitively* as a kid and I have exercised my entire adult life. In my early 20s, my relationship with exercise took a turn toward the compulsive. There was a period (about 5 years) where I exercised excessively as an intended means to counteract bouts of binge-eating. I refer to myself as a recovered exercise bulimic. Over-exercising never accomplished what I had hoped, and eventually I took other paths to address the causes of my binge-eating habits which were healthier and more successful.

But long after my personal exercise routine was right-sized, remnants of my unhealthy attitude toward exercise still lingered. For example, when I encountered another person who exercised the way I once did, I became uncomfortable …

almost threatened. I would question whether the frequency, duration, and intensity of my exercise routine was enough. I would feel *less than*. Conversely, I would sometimes self-righteously judge the other person who "hadn't seen the light yet." Both responses left me feeling off. Time after time, I gave away my serenity to this situation.

Eventually, a solution came to me. A yoga-loving friend of mine reminded me the meaning of the yoga expression namaste. This has worked perfectly ever since.

> Reflection:
> The fitness journey in me honors the fitness journey in you. Likewise, the successful aging journey in me honors the successful aging journey in you.

# 182

## Future Tripping & 4:30 p.m. Dinners: part 1

*Today is the first day* of my son's junior year in high school. To my delight, he still requested that I drive him to school. I did. I wasn't sure if I would cry, but I planned to let that be okay if it happened. I didn't. I deliberately planned to go directly to work after the drop-off. On my way to work, I made a couple of calls to mom friends. Then the tears began, but still not total weird-faced crying (which would have been okay, too). As always, I still cannot believe another year has gone by.

I love my work, and as soon as I arrived, I engaged my brain with thoughts about how best to serve my clients. I had written down my son's schedule, so in between clients I looked to see whether he was in physics, calculus, or US history at any given moment. I was doing fine. Then my last client left. It was just God, the dog and me. Here came the feelings and the Future Tripping. Here's what my head says when it is Future Tripping ….

"Well, he's begun his junior year of high school. Before you know it, he'll be graduating from high school and off to college. And you know what that means? Yup … he's as good as GONE right now! You might as well eat and eat a lot right now because this is gonna hurt like a MOFO and it will never stop hurting! And eating is the best solution." While all this chatter in my head continued, I ate the nutritious lunch I'd planned and contemplated adding more food to it.

I decided to call my friend Cordelia and leave her a voicemail. Her kids are in their 30s and we've talked about this issue before. Saying my feelings out loud helped ease the pain. I committed to her voicemail that I would postpone padding my food for 20 minutes while I completed a meditation app, lying down. I realized I wasn't sure if I was hungry or if I was only tired. I was sound asleep before the 20-minute guided meditation activity was over.

> Dear God,
> Help me remember that every feeling has a beginning, a middle, and an end. These sad feelings, too, shall pass.

# 183

## Future Tripping & 4:30 p.m. Dinners: Part II

*I awoke* from a 20-minute midday supine meditation/nap and wanted to eat again. I made a phone call to another friend. I was dubious she would even get where I was coming from, given she is only in her 30s and has no children. I explained to her how sad I was because my son might as well be gone already. Saying this out loud for the second time, and to someone so young, allowed me to hear the absurdity of my thinking. I was a little embarrassed. She seemed a little bored with my topic and moved on to another.

I committed to her I would not pad my food and would instead exercise in my home gym for 30 minutes. Long story short, I stuck to that commitment. Granted, I ate my dinner at 4:30 p.m., but I stuck to my plan and didn't pad my food.

My son has after-school activities, so I'll be picking him up at 6:00 p.m. today. One thing I know for sure: When I pick him up, I will be present and available for him because I haven't padded my food. When I began writing this book, my original motivation for not overeating was to avoid the Basketball. What I've learned along the journey is that while eating in moderation does help keep that basketball to a minimum, there is a much greater reward. When I eat to live, rather than live to eat, I am available for closer relationships with the ones I love. There is no better feeling in the world.

Boy, has this been one long day!

> Dear God,
> Give me the ability to stay in the present. And to remember I still have quite a while before my son moves out. If I spend my time wallowing in sadness and in the future, I'll miss the precious moments I still have with him.

# My Closing Thoughts

*You may not have a teenaged kid right now.* You may not even have kids. You may be perimenopausal. You may be post-menopausal or long beyond. You may be every color. Every height. Every size.

But whatever your situation, remember three things:

1. There are people in your life who want to connect with you. If you are eating beyond the point of feeling full, hopelessly preoccupied with dieting, compulsively shopping, drinking (or fill in the blank) to take the edge off, that will keep you from connecting and being available for them indefinitely.

2. You will experience feelings when your hormones shift. You will experience feelings for the rest of your life. They might not be as strong as mine. They might be much stronger. Let them come. Welcome them. Embrace them. They will pass and you will be better off for having embraced them. I promise. Whatever you are facing in your life right now, the power to overcome it is within you.

3. The world needs you to come out of isolation; loads of women want to connect with you to help destigmatize menopause and aging for generations to come. Now is the time!

You have so much more living to do. Join me in *Dammit volume 2,* where Cordelia and I will show you how we continue to age successfully one day at a time, with laughter, tears, and courage.

It's time to take this new, Varsity YOU out into the sunlight and make new contributions to the world.

Successful aging requires the acknowledgement of your extreme worth and potential in some small way, every day. *Dammit volume 2* builds on the Varsity Menopause successful aging foundation, and daily self-care techniques and then it goes deeper. I know it has taken a crap-ton of courage to get this far, but we're just getting started. *Dammit 2* goes deeper. More fear turned to courage, more tears and laughter, more love and more joy, more clarity and confidence … beyond your *wildest dreams!*

> *Take the time to invest in yourself.*
>
> *Make the life you dream of … the one you know you're meant to live … your Reality.*

*Are you ready to join me and an entire community of passionate women?*

*Are you ready to stop believing the lies your head tells you?*

*Are you ready to start the most inspired chapter of your life?*

*You're worth it!*
*You've got this!*
*We've got this!*

—Sally

# Acknowledgments

*Life doesn't just happen by itself.* Many have offered roadmaps and support through their written words and personal support. My Role Models/Teachers/Angels include:

1. Patricia Allen, PhD, Marriage & Family Therapist
2. Louise Hay; anything by her, but especially, *Life: Reflections on Your Journey* and *Heal Your Body*
3. Ann Corwin, PhD, MEd, Family and Child Development Consultant
4. Sandy McDaniel, Family and Child Development Consultant
5. Anne Lamott, Operating Instructions
6. Ellyn Satter, any book by her, but especially *Child of Mine: Feeding With Love* and *Good Sense*
7. Elizabeth Crary, any book by her, but especially *Dealing With Disappointment: helping kids cope when things don't go their way*

8. SARK (aka Susan Ariel Rainbow Kennedy), any book by her
9. Leila Zafaranchi, MD FACOG
10. Warren Cook
11. Miranda Nguyen
12. Melissa Pearl
13. Teresa Power
14. Monica
15. Beautiful H.
16. Baxter Bartlett

# About the Author

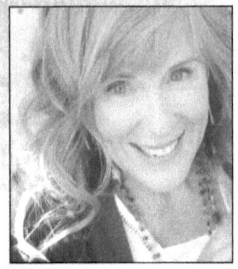

*Sally Bartlett* is an expert perimenopausal and menopausal coach, speaker and leader of women's online courses and retreats. She skillfully weaves together her academic and professional backgrounds with her decades-long personal experience of living in and loving the hell out of her right-sized body.

Sally earned a BA in psychology from UC Berkeley and is multi-certified by the American Council on Exercise, STOTT Pilates, and the MELT Method. For more than 20 years she has coached women aged 16-90 to reconnect with their bodies and to reignite their passion for movement with realistic expectations and radical self-acceptance.

Her Big Amazing Life resides in Southern California.

Coming Soon:
*Dammit ... It IS Menopause!*
*Companion Journal/Workbook*

# How to Work With Sally

## Online Courses:
### Level 1: The Healthy Body Mindset Recipe

Learn the Basic Ingredients for Body-Confidence in the 2nd Chapter of Your Life

Is your worth determined by your weight and your performance on your most recent diet? Do you yearn to put an end to self-loathing for the second chapter of your life, but don't know how? Develop a more current self-image with respect to aging, whether you have had body-confidence issues all your life or issues are just now arising for the first time with the onset of perimenopause. Break free from Diet Mentality.

- Identify negative self-talk that is holding you back.

- Learn a powerful journaling technique to redirect negative self-talk into positive self-talk in order to flourish.

- Find peace around food choices and freedom from dieting.

## Level 2: Finally Loving Your Body ... How To Maintain That!

Maintaining Your Body-Confidence Through Journaling.

Improve Emotional Regulation by getting current and staying current with your feelings. Learn new ways of living where you stay in touch with feelings and reignite and challenge your intellect. Are there some long-stifled passions inside just waiting to come out? Now is the time!

- Take a closer look at self-limiting beliefs and fears and negative self-talk.

- Expand on journaling strategies to develop and strengthen healthy self-talk.

- Cultivate an awareness of your actual passions that have been sabotaged by self-limiting beliefs time and time again.

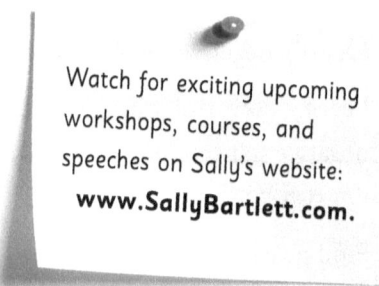

Watch for exciting upcoming workshops, courses, and speeches on Sally's website: **www.SallyBartlett.com.**

# Speaking Topics

### Dammit ... It IS Menopause ... Now What?

Are you not recognizing yourself in the mirror lately? Are you suddenly experiencing mood swings, hot flashes, forgetfulness and brain fog, to name a few?

- Why Your Life is So NOT Over.

- How to make a sustained daily commitment to living in and loving a healthy-sized body for optimal quality of life and aging.

- How to take the time to invest in yourself – and why you're worth it!

### It's Never too Late – Body-Confidence through Journaling: Imperfect Eating, Exercise, & Accountability

Do you have an inner critic that just won't quit? Learn how to use journaling techniques to acquaint yourself with a new, compassionate voice and rock your second chapter of life.

- Stop Dieting for good, learn self-compassion, and find peace.

- Learn how to stop the negative shame spiral when inevitable spontaneous eating occurs.
- Right-size your mindset around exercising for the purpose of disease prevention and healthy aging, cardiovascular health, muscle strength, bone strength, balance, fighting depression, sleeping better, pain-free movement, and adding to your energy levels.

To check on Sally's availability, call, or email:
**949-285-4212**
Sally@SallyBartlett.com
www.SallyBartlett.com

**Follow Sally on:**

- IamSallyBartlett
- @IamSallyBartlett
- @ImSallyBartlett
- Sally Bartlett
- IamSallyBartlett

# Now Available

**More Dammit ...
It IS Menopause!**
volume 2

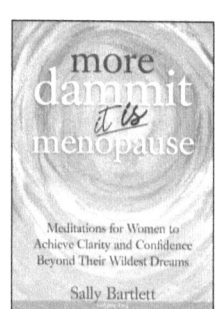

# Coming Soon

**Dammit ... It IS Menopause!**
Companion Journal / Workbook

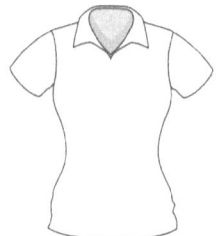

**Varsity Products:**
Varsity Transition T-shirts

www.ingramcontent.com/pod-product-compliance
Lightning Source LLC
Chambersburg PA
CBHW020900080526
44589CB00011B/376